FIRESIDE

THE
NAUTILUS

Ellington Darden, Ph.D.

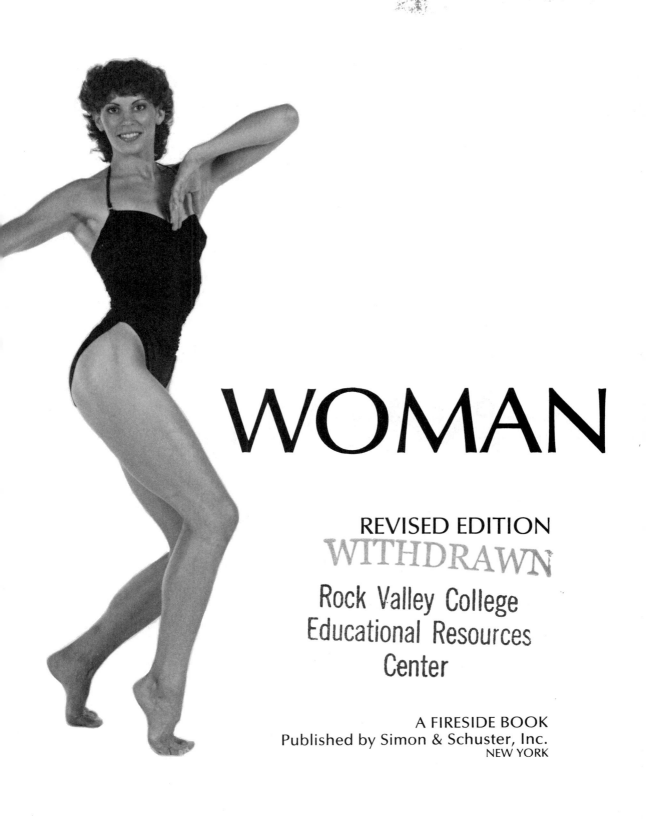

WOMAN

REVISED EDITION

A FIRESIDE BOOK
Published by Simon & Schuster, Inc.
NEW YORK

The Nautilus routines in this book are intended only for healthy women. Women with health problems should not follow the routines without a physician's approval. Before beginning any exercise program, always consult with your doctor.

BOOKS OF SPECIAL INTEREST TO WOMEN BY Ellington Darden, Ph.D.

Especially for Women
How to Lose Body Fat
The Superfitness Handbook
The Athlete's Guide to Sports Medicine
The Nautilus Nutrition Book
The Darden Technique for Weight Loss, Body Shaping, and
    Slenderizing
No More Fat!
The Nautilus Bodybuilding Book
The Nautilus Advanced Bodybuilding Book
The Nautilus Book
The Nautilus Diet

For a free catalog of Ellington Darden's fitness books, please send a self-addressed, stamped envelope to Darden Research Corporation, P.O. Box 1016, Lake Helen FL 32744.

Copyright © 1983, 1985 by Ellington Darden, Ph.D.

All rights reserved
including the right of reproduction
in whole or in part in any form

This Fireside Edition, 1986
Published by Simon & Schuster, Inc.
Simon & Schuster Building
Rockefeller Center
1230 Avenue of the Americas
New York, New York 10020

FIRESIDE and colophon are registered trademarks of Simon & Schuster, Inc.

Designed by Stanley S. Drate

Manufactured in the United States of America

10 9 8 7 6 5 4 3 2 1 Pbk.

Library of Congress Cataloging in Publication Data

Darden, Ellington
    The Nautilus woman.

    "A Fireside book."
    Bibliography: p.
    1. Weight lifting. 2. Exercise for women.
I. Title.
GV546.6.W64D37   1985   613.7'1   85-11962
ISBN 0-671-60034-6 Pbk.

Contents

Acknowledgments

I would like to thank the women who participated in the following parts of this book:

Susan Miller, 26, of Columbus, Ohio, for the artistic poses at the beginning of each chapter;

Mary Pluth, 28, of Orlando, Florida, for Chapter 5;

Pam Folsom D'Addio, 23, of Boca Raton, Florida, for Chapter 4 and Chapter 8;

Vi Folsom, 45, of Boynton Beach, Florida, for Chapter 10 and Chapter 11;

Shena Robinson, 20, of Orange City, Florida, for Chapter 7;

Susan Cunningham, 33, of Lake Helen, Florida, for Chapter 6 and Chapter 15;

Terri Jones, 21, of Lake Helen, Florida, for Chapter 9 and Chapter 12.

Lori Intelisano, 23, of Sanford, Florida, for appearing in the horizontal-striped leotard in five chapters and on the cover.

Special appreciation is extended to Estelle Cooper, Susan Cunningham, Robinette Thompson, and Susan Miller—all of whom read a draft of the manuscript and offered meaningful suggestions. Ken Hutchins assisted me in the writing of Chapter 2 and also reviewed the manuscript for technical accuracy. Ann Stewart turned my handwritten script into neatly typed pages.

The primary photography for the book was done by Robert Knorr. Ken Hutchins took the pictures of Lori Intelisano. Chris Lund contributed the photography in Chapter 14 and the front cover of Lori.

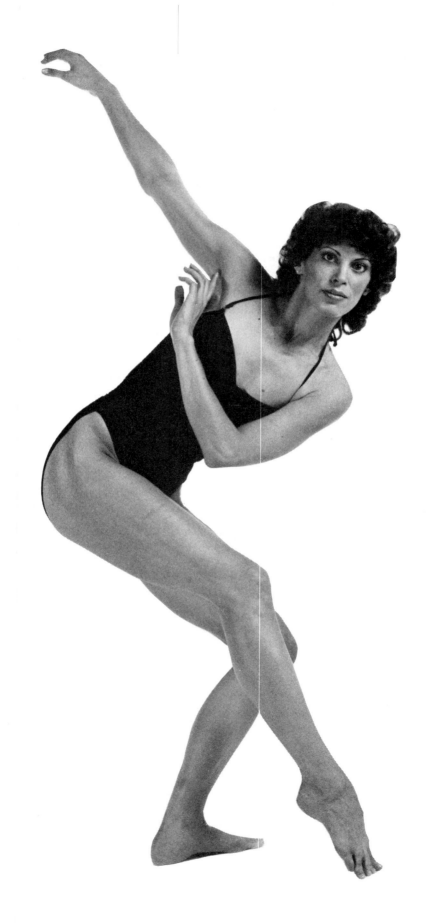

Preface

Approximately 54 percent of the adult population in the United States participate in exercise for body fitness, according to a Gallup Survey taken in November of 1984. This translates into nearly 92 million American adults.

An interesting revelation of these demographics is that women are much more likely to engage in exercise than men. Sixty percent of the fitness participants are female. Most importantly, however, men and women are discovering that strong, shapely biceps, triceps, pectorals, quadriceps, and hamstrings on the female frame can be healthy and sexy.

Twenty years ago, few women would venture into a gymnasium where men were lifting weights or "pumping iron." Today, in some areas of the country, there are as many women "pumping iron" as men.

When I first became associated with Nautilus Sports/Medical Industries in 1970, only a handful of women were attracted to our heavy-duty, steel-and-chrome exercise machines. But in 1986, there are numerous cities in the United States where more women are training on Nautilus equipment than men.

It is clear that women of the 1980's want more out of life. They want stronger muscles, greater endurance, and leaner bodies—and to be attractive at the same time. They want a no-nonsense approach to daily living. Nautilus provides the answer by manufacturing over 40 different exercise machines, many of which are specifically designed for women. Nautilus challenges women to reach their full potential, to become all they can become.

Nautilus-trained women are finding that they can take charge of the way they want their bodies to look. They can call their own shots when it comes to the strength and shape of their bodies.

For the last year, I have been training Terri Jones. Terri is featured in several chapters in this book. She writes a monthly article on women's fitness for the *Nautilus Magazine*. Her feelings about Nautilus training are stated below:

> Nautilus exercise has now become such an important part of my life that I don't feel normal when I miss my

regular workouts for a few days. In a very real sense I'm hooked on Nautilus.

Why? Because I've experienced life without Nautilus exercise. It just doesn't compare favorably with a daily routine that includes Nautilus. Until you've experienced life that includes proper exercise, there's no way you can judge the benefits.

Terri Jones understands the physical and psychological benefits of regular Nautilus exercise. She enjoys the positive contributions that Nautilus makes to her vibrant lifestyle.

Women today are also concerned with qualities that go beyond simply looking good, and Nautilus addresses some of these, too. Women have discovered that improved strength and endurance have helped them become more assertive and self-confident. These traits are instrumental in helping women attain greater success in both professional and personal fields.

The benefits of Nautilus training extend into many areas. But the basic benefit is simply that the woman who has gotten rid of her flaccid, flabby figure feels good about herself and her body. She is proud because she has done it on her own without help from plastic surgery.

The Nautilus Woman was written so all interested women could learn about the benefits of exercising on Nautilus equipment. It was also written to instruct women in how to get maximum results from each Nautilus machine.

This easy-to-understand book is divided into sixteen chapters. Chapter 1 introduces you to surprising research about physical attractiveness. You may discover the reasons behind some of your interpersonal behaviors.

Chapter 2 is about muscles. Do not casually skip over it. It may be the most important in the book because your muscles are the key to your body's beauty.

Chapter 3 provides you with detailed explanations of Nautilus training principles. You will want to read these guidelines several times.

Chapters 4–12 are presented in a how-to format. Each of your major body parts, from the calves up to the neck, is discussed. You will find all the necessary instructions and pictures on how to utilize each Nautilus machine for maximum efficiency.

Basic and specialized routines compose Chapter 13. Six basic routines are recommended for building an overall foundation of strength and fitness. The latter part of the chapter includes 17 specialized routines for attacking your problem areas, such as the thighs, hips, waist, arms, and chest.

Chapter 14 is especially for those women who are interested in competitive bodybuilding. The Nautilus routines described here will help any bodybuilder reach her goals faster.

Chapter 15 is designed for women who do not have regular access to Nautilus equipment. From this chapter, they should learn how to get the best bodyshaping results from freehand exercises.

The last chapter contains important fitness facts. Make certain you study it carefully. It answers the most frequently asked questions about Nautilus and exercise in general.

The most difficult part of Nautilus training is getting started. You have already taken the first step by reading the Preface. The other steps along the way are clearly marked in each chapter.

Congratulations. You are well on your way to becoming a Nautilus woman.

Ellington Darden, Ph.D.

Lake Helen, Florida

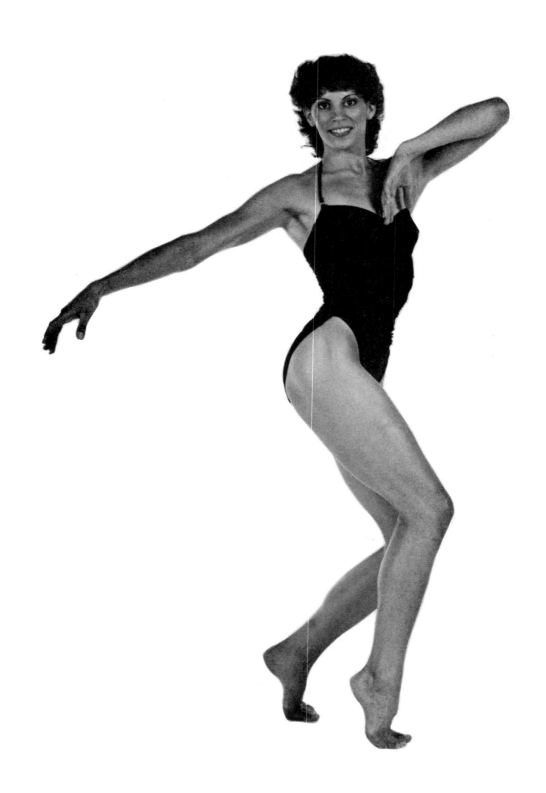

1

INTRODUCTION:
Body, Beauty, and Nautilus

What attracts a man to a woman? Is it her occupation? Her money? Her political beliefs? Or her personality?

No! It is the firm hips, slender legs, slim waist, and concave belly—or the shapely breasts, lean arms, and perfect posture that draw his attention.

Sigmund Freud noted 80 years ago that "anatomy is destiny . . . that attraction goes back to the physical."

Freud's belief has been repeatedly confirmed by Dr. Ellen Berscheid, professor of psychology at the University of Minnesota. Dr. Berscheid has been studying the effects of physical attractiveness for the last 15 years.

In a recent issue of *Psychology Today,* Dr. Berscheid and her colleague, Elaine Walster, reported a series of studies concerning college students involved in blind dating. What determined how well-liked the date was? Not exceptional personality features nor high intelligence, but, pure and simple, *physical attractiveness.*

Similar findings have been reported in connection with computer dating services. The main reason that most men asked for additional dates was physical beauty. Evidently, blind dates are blind to everything but appearance.

Importance of Physical Attractiveness

Are these findings really valid, since most dating is not of the blind or computer type? In order to answer a similar question, a survey was conducted by the *St. Petersburg Times.* The question, "What do boys like most about girls?" was circulated among the college students in that area of Florida. The results indicated that 79 percent of the answers dealt with something other than looks as most important.

Advice columnists Ann Landers and Abigail Van Buren would agree that looks are secondary in a relationship. They frequently downplay the physical and describe the ideal mate with such words as compassionate, dependable, honorable, forthright, gentle, loving, and forgiving.

Dr. Berscheid counters by saying that such beliefs come from parents and grandparents who taught us that it was vulgar to judge others by appearance. Such upbringing causes problems in many people who are naturally attracted to physical beauty, but then feel guilty afterward. What many of us are taught to believe and what is actually important to us are vastly different. "It is clearly a myth," says Berscheid, "that beauty is only skin deep. That our physical appearance should make an important difference in our lives is *not* a fact that makes most of us very comfortable."

A recent study by Dr. Eugene Mathes at Western Illinois University sheds even more light on the subject. Male and female college students were paired and asked to complete five dates with the same partners. Contrary to expectations, the study revealed that as the number of dates increased, physical attractiveness became a more important factor in determining if the partner was liked.

Dr. Berscheid says that the importance of physical attractiveness will continue to grow as increases in geographical mobility, frequent job changes, and divorce subject more people to one-time or few-time interactions with others. Such interactions force people to be judged on the basis of first impressions. Just as most people judge a book by its cover, they also form strong opinions of others from appearance alone.

Changing Our Appearance

"Genetic determinism is an anathema to Americans, who want to believe everyone is born equal," reports Dr. Berscheid. "It's simply not so! The most important factors governing success in life are genetically determined: height, sex, intelligence, and appearance."

All people are born with genes that determine their height, bone structure, eye color, sex, and intelligence. These are unalterable with one exception. Modern science has made possible sex change through surgery, but the individual who has this done cannot perform all the natural sex functions. Despite the fact that the above-mentioned factors are genetically unalterable, our appearance can be improved upon.

Our appearance is partially genetic and partially attained. Hair can be bleached or colored almost any shade. Specific clothes can be worn to hide a broad behind or a sagging belly. Cosmetic surgery can be used to remove unsightly blemishes, repair misaligned body parts, tighten wrinkled skin, and correct many other physical conditions. But the most practical, and many times the most efficient mode of altering the human body, is still *proper exercise.*

A clear distinction must be made between exercise for sport, recreation, or social endeavors and exercise for the purpose of toning, firming, and contouring the body. Recreational games and sporting activities are usually fun and enjoyable. But they rarely reach a level of intensity that would cause a physical change to occur. Exercise, in order to shape or reshape a woman's body, must be intense; and it must be progressive. Demanding, progressive exercise is not fun, but the results are striking and satisfying. In fact, the degree of firming and shaping of the body is directly related to the intensity of the exercise.

Nautilus Exercise

The most important advance in the history of high-intensity, progressive exercise occurred in 1970. That was the year Arthur Jones made available to the public his first Nautilus exercise machine. Jones was searching for ways to make exercise more intense—thus, more productive—and he succeeded.

Today, over 4.2 million people train on Nautilus machines throughout the United States: in high schools, colleges, sports-medicine clinics, training rooms, athletic clubs, health spas, and in over 4,000 Nautilus Fitness Centers. "Reports show that 50 percent of the members of Nautilus Fitness Centers are women," says Jim Flanagan, general manager of Nautilus Sports/Medical Industries, "and the percentage of women is increasing every month."

In order for exercise to shape a woman's body, specific muscles must be isolated, then stretched and contracted against resistance throughout a full range of possible movement. Nautilus machines are specifically designed according to the physiological functions of the human body. Nothing is more effective at bodyshaping than Nautilus.

So if you are interested in slimming your hips, thighs, and waist, firming your buttocks and arms, and shaping your calves and breasts, simply apply the concepts in this book. And the next time someone tells you, "I like your legs," or "You have a beautiful waistline," or even "I love your body," you can believe him!

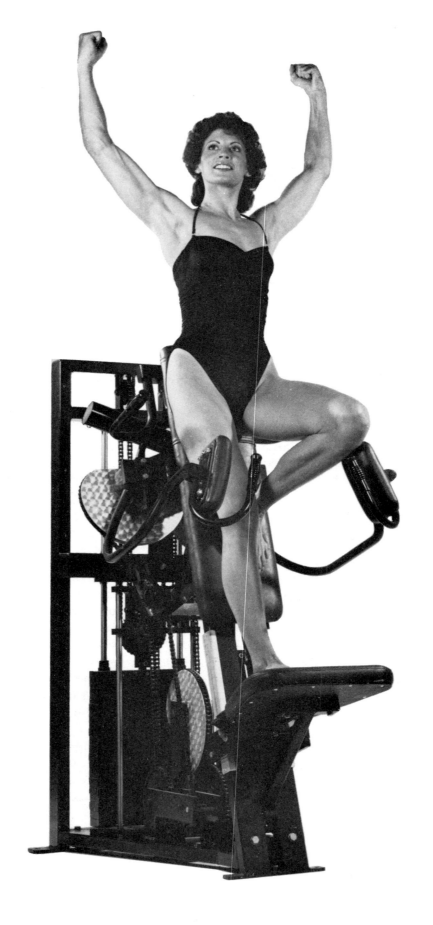

2
MUSCLES:
Conquering the Fears

Women traditionally have had numerous fears about their muscles. Let us eavesdrop on a typical conversation that might occur almost anywhere women get together.

"Weight training develops large, masculine muscles," says one woman in defense of why she does not want to participate in strenuous exercise.

"I'm all for stretching movements," says another woman, "since stretching produces long, smooth, flexible muscles. Besides, everyone knows that lifting weights makes you bulky and tight."

"Training your muscles makes you gain weight," says a middle-aged housewife. "I want to lose weight, not gain it."

"Muscles most definitely are for men, not women," notes another figure-conscious lady.

"But you know," says an attractive woman, "I keep reading articles about Bo Derek, Farrah Fawcett, Jane Fonda, and other movie stars who swear by heavy exercise. How could these movie stars look so beautiful and be so wrong?"

Are Bo Derek, Farrah Fawcett, and Jane Fonda really wrong about the connection between vigorous exercise and good looks? Or are the traditional fears that many women share about training their muscles based on myths and superstitions? A scientific examination of these concepts will help to separate the facts from the fallacies.

Developing Large Muscles

Most women believe that if they participate in weight training, they will build large, unfeminine muscles. But it is virtually impossible for a woman to develop excessively large muscles.

Building large muscles requires two factors. First, the individual must have long muscle bellies and short tendon attachments. Second, an adequate amount of male hormones, particularly testosterone, must be present in the bloodstream. Women seldom have long muscle bellies; in fact, this is even rare among men. And women have less than one-hundredth the amount of testosterone in their blood than do men.

Research studies comparing the body composition changes of college-age males and females following a weight-training program have been reported in several scientific journals by Dr. Jack Wilmore of the University of California at Davis. Dr. Wilmore concluded that while weight training increases the muscle mass in both the male and female, it is much less pronounced in the female. The largest increase in muscular girth (circumference) exhibited by the females was only 0.6 centimeter—or less than a quarter of an inch! Such small increases in girth clearly indicate that muscular growth in the female as a result of weight-training programs will not lead to bulky muscles or produce a masculinizing effect.

This very small increase in the circumference measurement of a trained body part—the upper thigh, for example—may appear to be the reason some women feel that their pants are fitting tighter around their thighs. The real reason, however, is a phenomenon known as "heightened perception of touch." Heightened perception of touch means that a person becomes more aware of a particular body part (the skin surrounding the thighs, in this instance) because of the increased blood flow, strength, and firmness of the underlying muscles as a result of regular and concentrated exercise. Because of correct exercise, the previously dormant parts of her thighs have become more sensitive and alive. This muscular sensation is also transferred to the surrounding tissues. Her pants feel tighter, not because they are tighter, but because she can now, perhaps for the first time in her life, perceive the material next to her skin. This phenomenon can also occur in other parts of a woman's body such as the hips, back, shoulders, and arms.

The inability of women to develop bulky muscles has been repeatedly confirmed by long-term research projects conducted on female cadets at the United States Military Academy at West Point and by ongoing research with women at the Nautilus Research Clinic in Lake Helen, Florida. Proper weight training has always, with virtually no exceptions, improved the physical attractiveness of every female trainee.

Yet, almost every woman has seen pictures of women who do have unusually large muscles. These large-muscled women are products of their genes rather than products of an exercise program.

They have inherited above-average-length muscles and above-average levels of male hormones; thus the ability to develop larger and more defined muscles than the typical woman. These few women, whether they exercise or take part in sports or not, will be larger and stronger than the average woman. But only one in a million women would fall into this category.

If a woman who had all the genetic capabilities actually did develop unsightly muscles, she could go without exercise for a week and her muscles would shrink. Muscles are made to be used, and if they are not, they decrease in size.

Importance of Muscle

The basic confusion that women most commonly experience is directly related to misinformation regarding the actual properties of muscle. Muscle contributes both to a woman's outside appearance and to her overall physical fitness.

Muscle, and only muscle, produces movement of the body. Other factors contribute to and are necessary for organized movement to occur, but only the muscles produce the contractile forces necessary to propel the body of any woman or man. To increase the size and strength of the musculature serves to make human movement more secure and efficient.

Muscle also serves to protect the body from physical harm. Not only does a stronger muscle enable a woman to move more efficiently, but joint stability is dependent on the dynamic muscular force about each joint. Growing muscles directly and indirectly increase the strength of the connective tissues, tendons, ligaments, and bone.

But what about appearance? It is well documented that feminine curves are the result of female fat distribution initiating with puberty and continuing throughout the teenage years. These curves are cosmetically appealing as long as they are well supported by the underlying muscle and do not have an excessive number of fat cells. Sagging fat is not appealing. Fat is feminine and appealing only when it is firm and properly distributed. Most women's figure problems are related to the condition of being undermuscled and overfat simultaneously.

Since an overfat condition plagues many women, an increase in muscle serves another valuable purpose. Muscle is the foremost consumer of energy in the body. When the quantity and strength of a woman's muscles are increased, more fuel is required to sustain them at work and at rest. Her basal metabolism will increase and this will supplement the impact of a low-calorie diet.

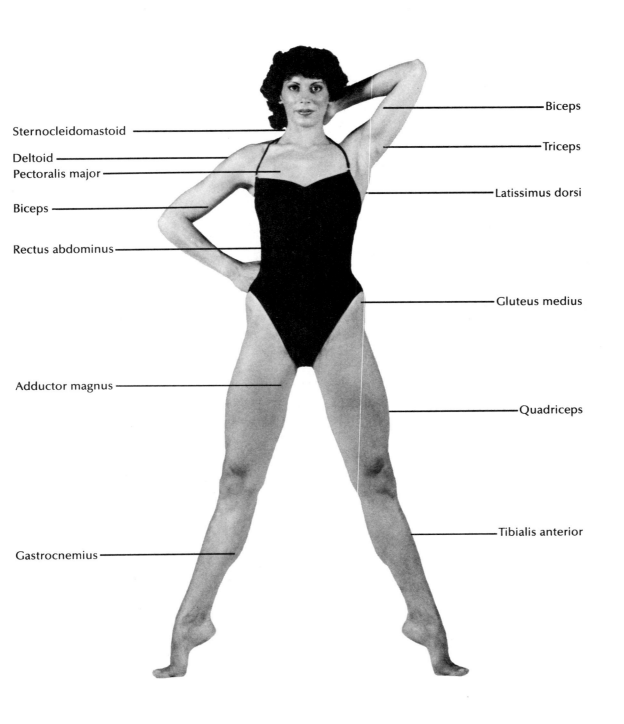

Sternocleidomastoid ——————————

Deltoid ——————

Pectoralis major ——————

Biceps ——————

Rectus abdominus ——————

Adductor magnus ——————

Gastrocnemius ——————

Biceps ——————

Triceps ——————

Latissimus dorsi ——————

Gluteus medius ——————

Quadriceps ——————

Tibialis anterior ——————

Major Muscles of a Woman's Body—
FRONT VIEW

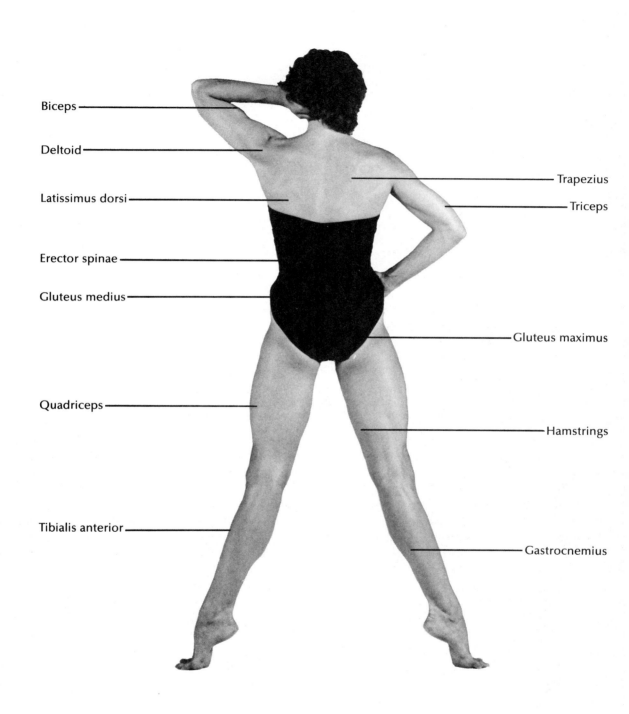

Biceps

Deltoid

Latissimus dorsi

Erector spinae

Gluteus medius

Quadriceps

Tibialis anterior

Trapezius

Triceps

Gluteus maximus

Hamstrings

Gastrocnemius

Major Muscles of a Woman's Body—
BACK VIEW

Proper exercise, therefore, has a double-reducing effect on a woman's body. First, it burns calories during the actual exercise. Second, it leads to stronger muscles that are significantly more calorie-demanding for the body to maintain. Stronger muscles can help a woman lose body fat and keep it off.

Also, muscular strength and endurance are important during pregnancy. Many of the negative aspects of pregnancy, both cosmetic deterioration and labor difficulties, are the result of weak muscles. Proper exercise for a pregnant woman is probably more important than at any other time of her life.

Thus far, the facts reveal that Bo Derek, Farrah Fawcett, and Jane Fonda are right. There is a definite connection between vigorous exercise and good looks. High-intensity exercise will transform a woman's important body parts into firmer and more shapely flesh.

A selection of popular women's magazines that have promoted vigorous exercise for a more attractive body.

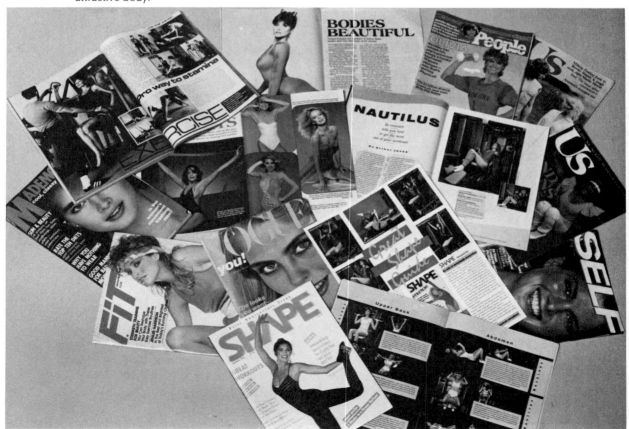

Stretching Movements and Flexibility

For years, stretching movements have been used almost as a cure-all. Women have been told that stretching will improve their flexibility, firm and shape their body, reduce fat, and prevent injuries. As a result, women by the thousands stretch their bodies in organized classes at local clubs or in front of television instructors at home, with and without various types of music.

Most women are attracted to stretching movements simply because they are easy, fun, and social, especially since large groups can be directed in the same movements in unison. This is certainly acceptable. But the facts show that the potential physiological benefits from stretching programs are vastly overrated and indeed limited.

Stretching performed slowly and smoothly does improve a person's flexibility. Flexibility is defined as the range of movement of a body segment around a joint or group of joints. Women, because of their hormones and body composition, are generally more flexible than men. This is especially true of a woman's lower body. Yet most women seem to concentrate on movements that stretch the muscles of their hips and thighs. They mistakenly believe that stretching strengthens and firms their muscles, which it does not; that stretching lengthens their muscles, which it does not; or that stretching reduces the fatty deposits on their hips and thighs, which it does not.

Furthermore, there are no conclusive data that increased flexibility prevents injuries. Too much flexibility, in fact, can cause injuries. What research does show is that muscular strength throughout full-range joint movement is the primary factor that prevents injury.

Women need to emphasize proper strength training much more than stretching movements. It is the strength of the muscles, not the flexibility of the joints, that contributes to a shapely figure.

Body Weight or Body Fat?

Another source of misinformation is centered on the bathroom scales. For generations, American mothers have led their daughters to the bathroom to take a reading on the trusty scales. Information acquired from beauty parlors, social clubs, and glamour magazines perpetuates and reinforces the idea that a woman's appearance depends on her body weight.

If you have ever taken a basic chemistry course, you are probably familiar with the terms "qualitative analysis" and "quantitative analysis." When the chemistry instructor provides an unknown to solve, he might request a quantitative analysis. He will provide you information concerning what you are analyzing, but he wants you to measure its quantity.

Yet, if the instructor requests a qualitative analysis, he is asking the chemistry student to provide the "what." In other words, you must tell him the name of the substance measured.

Body weight is quantitative. It is entirely meaningless for a woman to refer to her weight as, for instance, 110 pounds without stating its qualities. What weights 110 pounds? Fat? Muscles? Bones? Salt? Lead? Corn flakes? All of the above? And if so, then in what proportions? What weighs 110 pounds?

It should be perfectly clear that weight signifies nothing. Body weight is irrelevant. The words "body weight," "overweight," and "underweight" should be removed from all fitness magazines and books. It is not a factor of health and well-being. Concern should be placed on the body's degree of fatness.

"Lose 10 pounds in a week. Order today!"

How many times have you read such claims in beauty magazines? Such phrases steer women into believing that there is a quick and easy method to fat loss when the advertisements really mean weight loss. This is merely a misleading advertisement that tells women what they desperately want to hear. The truth is that you can lose only 3 to 4 ounces of fat per day and know that it is fat. If any more weight than that amount is lost, then the weight is something other than fat: something a woman should retain, such as fluid from her blood and muscles.

Even if a woman follows a sensible fat-reduction diet, she often fails to combine it with proper exercise. After several weeks she is smaller and lighter. She is also weaker, lethargic, more prone to injury, and shapeless with poor posture. She has reduced herself to a virtual bag of bones. In order to prevent the wasting away of muscle mass, a strength-training program must accompany a fat-reduction diet so that a woman increases or at least maintains her muscle mass.

A Possible Course of Events

Kathy, age 24, recently joined a Nautilus Fitness Center. The staff told her they could provide the fastest, safest method to increase her strength and endurance, enhance her figure, and reduce her fat. She adhered to the prescribed program of high-intensity exercise combined with a low-calorie diet. After the first two weeks she felt better than she had in many years.

On Monday morning of the seventh week, however, Kathy stopped by to register complaints with her training consultant. She was considering quitting her exercises. Why was Kathy experiencing misgivings about the program?

Most of her discontent was due to the misunderstandings regarding exercise and fat loss already discussed. These erroneous beliefs were destroying her motivation and patience. They were compounded by emotional and social factors that she was not able to identify. What was causing the misgivings that Kathy was experiencing?

First, some of the most disciplined trainees begin to lose motivation at about the sixth week. Kathy's proficiency on Nautilus equipment was beginning to have a profound effect—the intensity of the exercise was becoming very demanding. Of course, this was desirable for the best possible physical benefits, but as the exercise becomes more difficult, the novelty wears off.

Second, Kathy was receiving advice—bad advice. During her six weeks of membership, she had been to church four times, to three different parties, visited her mother twice, her grandparents once, and talked of her Nautilus experience with them—and also her boss, her new boyfriend, and all her co-workers. In jest, Kathy's boyfriend and boss had asked to feel her biceps, and jokingly asked if she aspired to be a woman bodybuilder. Partly because they saw no harm in making her the butt of their jokes, and partly because exercise may still be viewed as a male domain, her boss and boyfriend had actually been very destructive to her program. They might even have been jealous of her; jealous that they were not enrolled, and that a woman was in their rightful place. For lack of anything intelligent to say, they seized the opportunity to crush what little confidence she had about her program.

Third, Kathy saw a women's bodybuilding contest on television. She wrongly assumed that if a gathering of 25 muscular women can be viewed in one location simultaneously, there must be thousands of women experiencing the same result from strength training. Little did she realize that such women are rare genetic specimens who were posing for a camera lens that distorts their size even further. Their attributes reinforced her fear of the muscular strength she desperately needed.

Fourth, Kathy possibly had tried passive figure salons, body wraps, or spot-reduction clinics, all of which are high-pressure consumer frauds. Her family skeptically suggested that "Kathy has done it again." They may have grudgingly resented that she had joined a Nautilus facility because they believed she would be ripped off once more.

Fifth, an area of specialized attention for Kathy had been her flabby hips and thighs. She used the Nautilus hip and thigh machines for strengthening these problem areas. As her muscles strengthened

Rock Valley College - ERC

they became slightly larger. They also grew firmer, smoothing the dimpled fatty deposits—erroneously termed "cellulite"—to give her a shapely, graceful contour. The realization that muscle "strength" and muscle "size" are closely related may have frightened Kathy. She had never encountered high-intensity exercise and initially a woman's muscles may respond more quickly than a man's.

Sixth, Kathy wore well-tailored clothes. They seemed to fit differently, especially about the hips and thighs. Her figure was dramatically improved in some areas, but her clothes appeared to fit tighter at the hips and along the upper thighs. Nautilus training had given Kathy "heightened perception of touch" in her lower body. The circumference of her hips and thighs was not larger. It simply felt that way because of her skin's improved sensitivity.

Before a woman's major fat deposits will show a decrease in size, she must diligently adhere to her low-calorie diet for several weeks, perhaps months. Kathy had to remember that only a few ounces of fat per day, or a little more than a pound of fat per week can be lost. This loss will be from fat stored throughout her body, not just from a particular area where she focuses her exercise attention. Spot reducing is impossible.

Pinch up a fold of skin from the back of your hand, the side of your waist, and the front of your thigh. Notice the comparative thicknesses between your fingers. If a reduction, say 10 percent, of the fat throughout the body is made, each of these areas will reduce proportionately 10 percent. But which of the three will be noticeably smaller? The larger fat deposit, at the waist or thigh, will appear smaller; the back of the hand will be unnoticed. Nevertheless, 10 percent of the fat from the back of the hand and throughout the body will be lost.

Note that the Nautilus staff promised Kathy that she would "reduce fat." What she heard was "reduce weight." So when six weeks later, Kathy weighed a few pounds more, she was disturbed and started to panic. The staff may have failed to explain to her that muscle is denser than fat. A very obese woman should certainly lose weight as she reduces fat and adds muscle, but many women will become heavier as they become slimmer, leaner, and stronger. Actual weight is meaningless.

There you have it: six reasons for Kathy's misgivings about her Nautilus program which had, in fact, brought very positive results. The problem was lack of interpretation. But who should Kathy believe? Should she take the word of a Nautilus instructor or listen to the input from family, friends, television, beauty magazines, and the fears made real to her by the changes she sees in her body? Kathy was frightened and the Nautilus instructor was outnumbered. How could he win her confidence?

Perhaps the best method to combat Kathy's or other women's fears is to address them before they are experienced. Fears can be conquered with scientific facts, scientific facts which are understood and applied. Education, quality education, remains the best way to conquer fears about high-intensity exercise.

Victory Close at Hand

Most women will experience many of the foregoing events. They collectively represent the ultimate obstacle for a woman's training program. If she can weather this experience, she will begin to realize the possible benefits that high-intensity exercise bestows. She will become the easiest trainee to supervise; she will perform the exercise in better form than most of her male counterparts, and will achieve desirable results that serve to reinforce her motivation beyond her own imagination. Within six months she will be leaner, firmer, healthier, and sexier. She will be more feminine and beautiful, and she will have more endurance and less susceptibility to injury. Her enthusiasm will be high because she understands.

At the onset of her high-intensity program a woman is unsure and frightened. She does not yet truly believe in the regimen because of minimal acquaintance with Nautilus exercise. Properly instructed a woman slowly begins to understand as well as believe in her program.

When a woman intelligently hurdles the major obstacles described in this chapter, she is well on her way toward reaping the maximum benefits of Nautilus training.

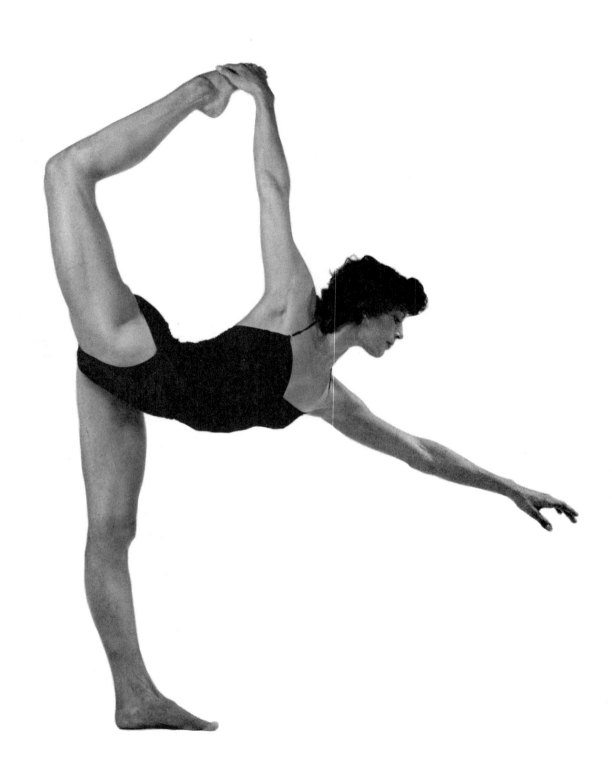

3
PRINCIPLES:
Isolation and Intensity

Nautilus Sports/Medical Industries was founded to develop and manufacture exercise equipment that builds body shape, strength, endurance, and flexibility.

Nautilus equipment is based on thorough research into the precise function of each muscle group, from full stretch to complete contraction. It is designed to exercise the muscular structure through this full range of movement with proportional resistance on an automatically adjusting basis. This automatically adjusting resistance is primarily a result of the patented Nautilus cam, which is incorporated into every machine. A Nautilus cam is a scientifically designed pulley with an off-center axis. Since the profile of one of the early cams resembled the silhouette of the chambered nautilus shell, the revolutionary machines were given the same name.

The science behind every Nautilus machine is isolation and exercise of specific muscle groups with correct form and method. Application of this concept is an essential component in the design of any exercise device.

The first Nautilus-type machine was built in 1948, and after 22 years of further research and development, the equipment was finally perfected and produced for sale.

The unique idea on which Nautilus is founded was not available until the equipment was developed and ready for use. Before Nautilus, the basic tools for conditioning were calisthenics or free-hand movements, gymnastic bars, barbells, dumbbells, cables and pulleys, spring devices, and friction machines. Such tools had remained virtually unchanged in concept and application for over 50 years. In the 1970's, Nautilus machines began to make a significant

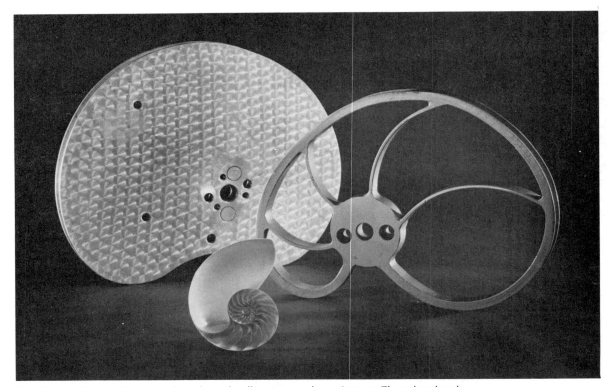

The first Nautilus machines used steel spiral pulleys to vary the resistance. These handmade spiral pulleys or cams resembled the cross section of a nautilus shell. Today, the Nautilus cams are shaped from solid block aluminum to scientific specifications by a profile milling machine.

impact on the training and conditioning habits of fitness-minded Americans. It only took one Nautilus workout to convince most trainees that Nautilus was something special. Soon the revolution was on.

The reason Nautilus revolutionized conditioning was, in one word, *efficiency.* Nautilus training was much more efficient than traditional methods. Earlier methods of conditioning had centered on long programs of exercise. To obtain a high level of fitness, an individual had to spend a minimum of 90 minutes a day on stretching for flexibility, jogging for heart-lung endurance, and lifting barbells for muscular strength and shape. The average fitness enthusiast might spend from 5 to 10 hours a week on such a variety of programs.

Best Possible Results

If Nautilus machines required the same amount of time as traditional methods and produced slightly better results, that would still be a worthwhile contribution. But if Nautilus machines produced three times the results in only a fraction of the time, that could only be described as revolutionary. That is exactly what Nautilus produced: three times the results in a fraction of the time.

What does this mean if you are an average fitness-minded or figure-conscious woman? Simply that when you use Nautilus equipment properly, you will be getting the best possible results.

Thousands of women, however, spend untold time exercising on Nautilus equipment without having a sound understanding of how to use each machine properly. Although they are getting some results, the results are not what they should be.

Assume that an average woman has the potential of getting 100 units of results in six months from each Nautilus machine. Training regularly for six months, she obtains 25 units of improvement. Some women will be satisfied with such benefits; other women will be disappointed. Regardless of the feelings, both groups could be getting two, three, or even four times better results if they had a clear understanding of how best to use each piece of Nautilus equipment.

Intensity of Exercise

The simplest, most rapid method of achieving physical transformation involves high-intensity exercise. High intensity means performing an exercise to the point of momentary muscular failure; a point reached when it is temporarily impossible to achieve another repetition properly.

High-intensity exercise mobilizes the greatest amount of muscle mass. Muscle mass is composed of many fibers. Low-intensity work uses only some of those fibers. High-intensity Nautilus training uses the maximum amount possible.

An exercise on most Nautilus machines should be performed for 8 to 12 repetitions. If you cannot do 8, the resistance is too heavy. If you can do more than 12, the resistance is too light. It should be increased at the next workout.

Many of the popular activities in women's classes aim at reaching hundreds of repetitions with low-intensity exercises. Regardless of the number of repetitions performed, low-intensity work can never approach the benefits of high-intensity work.

High-intensity training on Nautilus equipment must be brief and infrequent. Long workouts may actually result in a loss of strength and condition. This is another advantage of Nautilus exercise: besides being more efficient, it is a time saver.

Correct form should be practiced on each machine. Every repetition should be performed in a smooth, steady manner throughout the full range of possible movement. Special attention should be given to the lowering, or negative portion of each repetition. Negative exercise is described on pages 175–77.

Bodyshaping Guidelines

It has taken Nautilus Sports/Medical Industries many years of research and testing to establish the following bodyshaping principles for women:

1. Perform approximately 4 to 6 exercises for the lower body and 6 to 8 exercises for the upper body, and no more than 12 exercises in any workout.

2. Train no more than three times a week. High-intensity Nautilus exercise necessitates a recovery period of at least 48 hours. The body gets stronger during rest, not during exercise.

3. Select a resistance for each exercise that allows the performance of between 8 to 12 repetitions.

   (a) Begin with a weight you can comfortably do 8 times. The lightest weight on any Nautilus machine is 20 pounds, which includes a single top plate and the vertical selector rod. Some machines have double top plates, so the lightest possible weight on them is 30 pounds. Each additional plate weighs 10 pounds.

   (b) Stay with that weight until 12 or more strict repetitions are performed. On the following workout, increase the resistance by approximately 5 percent. *Note:* 5 percent of a beginning weight, such as 20 pounds, is only 1 pound. Nautilus is now manufacturing small saddle plates weighing 1¼, 2½, 5, and 7½ pounds which, when correctly added onto the top plate of a machine, will allow you to progress in a systematic manner.

   (c) Attempt constantly to increase the number of repetitions or the amount of weight, or both. But do not sacrifice form in an attempt to produce repetition and resistance improvements.

4. Keep accurate records—date, resistance, repetitions, and overall training time—of each workout.

5. Position the body correctly on all single-joint rotary machines. The axis of the Nautilus cam should be in line with the joint of the body part that is being exercised.

When you can perform 12 or more repetitions on a Nautilus machine, that is the signal to increase the resistance by 5 percent at the next workout. This progression in resistance is best accomplished by the addition of small saddle plates.

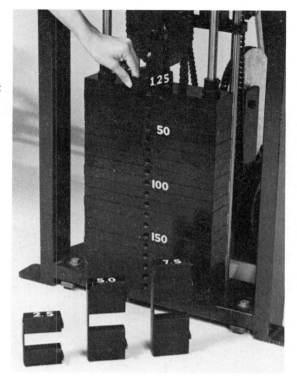

6. Maintain the body in a properly aligned position on each machine. Avoid twisting or shifting the torso and trunk during the last repetitions.

7. Concentrate on stretching by moving slowly during the first three repetitions of each exercise.

8. Accentuate the lowering or negative portion of each repetition. Lift the resistance smoothly in 2 seconds and lower it slowly in 4 seconds.

9. Move slower, never faster, if in doubt about the speed of movement.

10. Do everything possible to isolate and work each large muscle group to exhaustion.

11. Relax body parts that are not involved in each exercise. Pay special attention to relaxing the face and hand muscles.

12. Breathe normally. Try not to hold your breath during any repetition.

For maximum benefits from Nautilus training, the 12 bodyshaping principles must be combined with a knowledge of how to use specific Nautilus machines. The next nine chapters describe and illustrate the correct use of Nautilus machines, body part by body part.

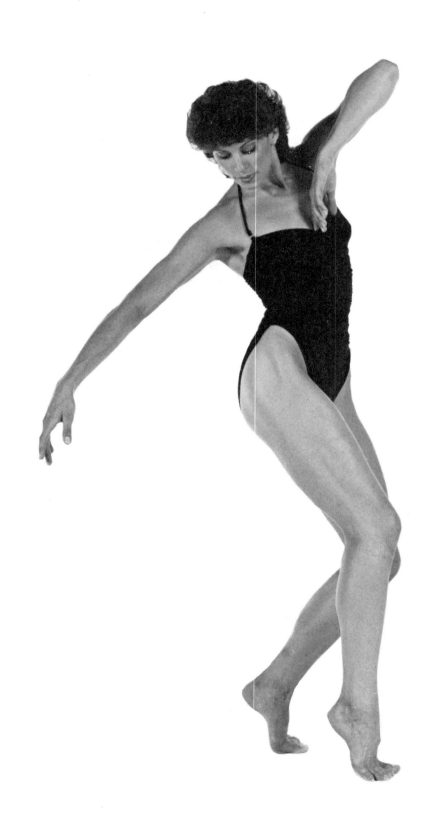

4
HIPS:
Fighting Those Lumps and Bumps

"Standing on the corner watching all the girls go by," echoes the familiar song of the 1950's.

Girl-watching is a popular pastime that is enjoyed by men as well as women—whether it be on a street corner, in an airport, or on a sandy beach. Furthermore, people enjoy watching people watch each other.

One of the real turn-offs, from a girl-watcher's perspective, is to see flabby hips and buttocks oozing from tight shorts, jeans, or a bathing suit.

Besides looking awful in a swimsuit and most other clothes, a bulgy backside also results in poor carriage and an ungraceful stride. Much of the muscle power used to walk, run, and support the spinal column stems directly from the gluteal muscles of the buttocks.

There are three gluteal muscles, and they are named according to their size. The gluteus maximus is the largest and overlies the other two muscles. Broad and thick, the gluteus maximus gives the buttocks their characteristic rounded shape. The primary function of this muscle is to move the thigh from a stretched position with the knee close to the chest, to a contracted position with the thigh behind the torso. You can feel the gluteus maximus muscles contract when you climb stairs.

On the opposite side of the gluteus maximus are the iliopsoas muscles of the frontal hip area. The iliopsoas flex the hip or move the thighs forward.

The other two gluteal muscles, the gluteus medius and gluteus minimus, are located on the outer surface of the hipbone. Movement of one thigh away from the other, called hip abduction, is the major function of these two muscles.

The hips and buttocks should be smooth, curved, and well-toned. Flabby weak gluteals tend to sag, which in turn causes the overlying fat to have an orange-peel look. Saddlebags soon form on the outer hips as well. Much of this flabbiness, however, can be remedied with proper use of three Nautilus machines: duo hip and back, hip flexion, and hip abduction. The gluteals can be toned, smoothed, and shaped. Only Nautilus provides full-range, direct exercise for fighting those unslightly lumps and bumps on your backside.

Duo Hip and Back Machine

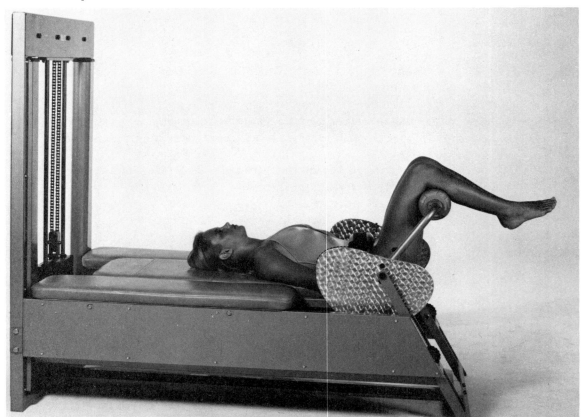

Muscles used: gluteus maximus, erector spinae, and hamstrings
Points to emphasize:
1. Enter machine from front by separating movement arms.
2. Lie on back with both legs over roller pads.
3. Align hip joint with axes of cams.
4. Fasten seat belt and grasp handles lightly. Seat belt should be snug, but not too tight, as back must be arched at completion of movement.

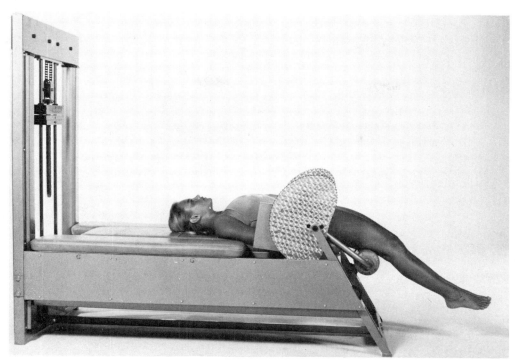

5. Extend both legs and at the same time push back with arms. With a heavy weight, extend one leg and hold it in the down position. Extend the other leg to the same position.

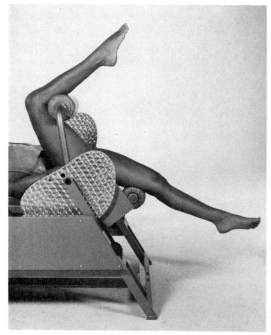

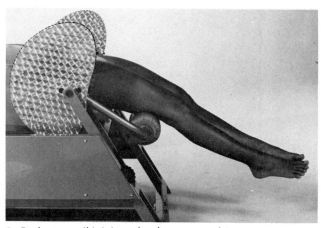

8. Push out until it joins other leg at extension.
9. Pause, arch lower back, and contract buttocks. In contracted position, keep legs straight, knees together, and toes pointed.
10. Repeat with other leg and continue alternating one leg with the other.

6. Keep one leg at full extension. Allow other leg to bend and come back as far as possible.
7. Stretch.

Hip Flexion Machine

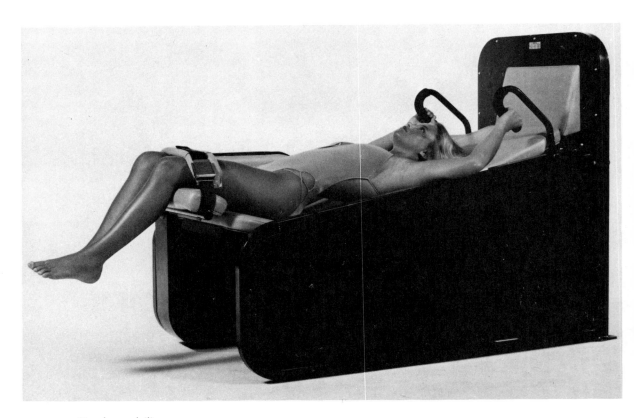

Muscle used: iliopsoas
Points to emphasize:
1. Sit in machine.
2. Fasten seat belt across thighs.
3. Lie back in reclining position.
4. Grasp handles by head.
5. Keep torso and head on seat back.

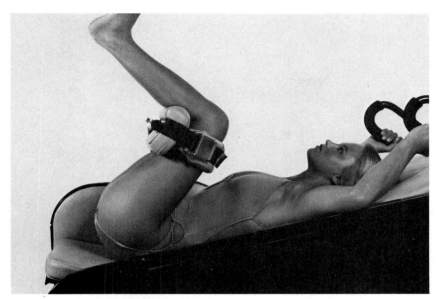

6. Flex hips smoothly by drawing knees to chest.
7. Pause.

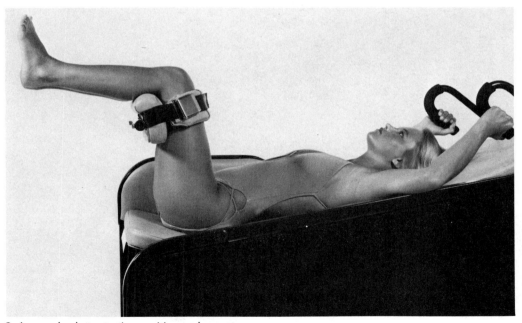

8. Lower slowly to starting position and repeat.

Hip Abduction Machine

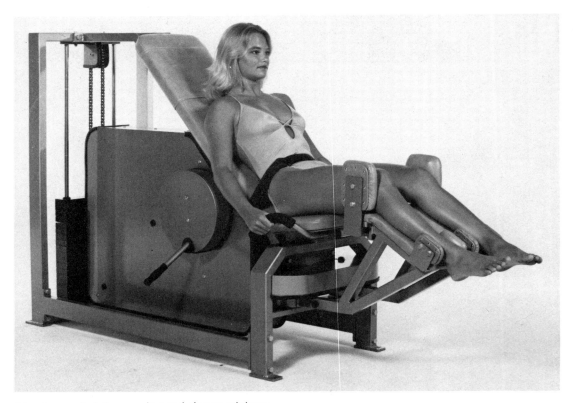

Muscles used: gluteus medius and gluteus minimus
Points to emphasize:
1. Sit in machine and place legs on movement arms. Some women may require an extra back pad.
2. Fasten seat belt.
3. Keep head and shoulders against seat back.

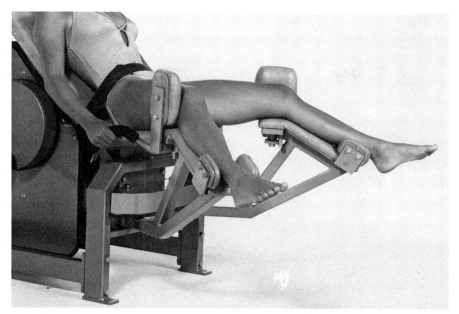

4. Push knees and thighs laterally to widest position.
5. Pause.

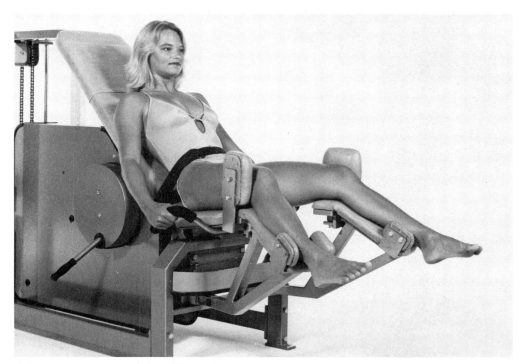

6. Return to knees-together position and repeat.

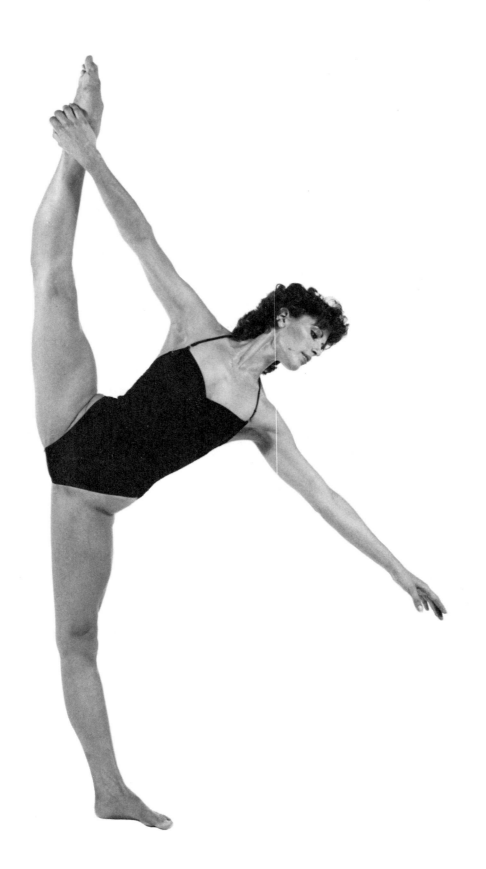

5
THIGHS:
Long and Lean

Women of all ages complain about their thighs. Their outer thighs are dimpled. Their inner thighs are like jelly. Their back thighs lack contour. They have puffiness over their kneecaps. Out-of-shape muscles, no matter where they occur, most often result from lack of high-intensity exercise. Regular Nautilus exercise will make your legs appear longer and leaner.

Most women want to improve their thighs for cosmetic reasons. Strengthening these muscles will also protect the knee, the most vulnerable joint in the body. The knee bears 85 percent of the body's weight. It is frequently injured in sports and fitness activities, as well as normal responsibilities around the home. Toning and shaping the thigh muscles will help stabilize this vital joint.

The major muscles of the front and back thighs are the quadriceps and hamstrings. When the quadriceps muscles contract the leg straightens. The hamstrings muscles bend the leg.

The medial or inner thighs are composed of a third set of muscles, the adductor group. Contraction of these muscles brings the thighs from a spread-legged to a knees-together position. This movement is called hip adduction.

Training the thighs on Nautilus will most definitely improve the figure. Heavy thighs can be slimmed. Thin thighs can be strengthened and shaped to look more attractive. Disproportional thighs can be exercised to become more symmetrical. With the Nautilus thigh machines, you do not have to settle for anything less than long, lean, lithe thighs.

Compound Leg Machine, Leg Extension

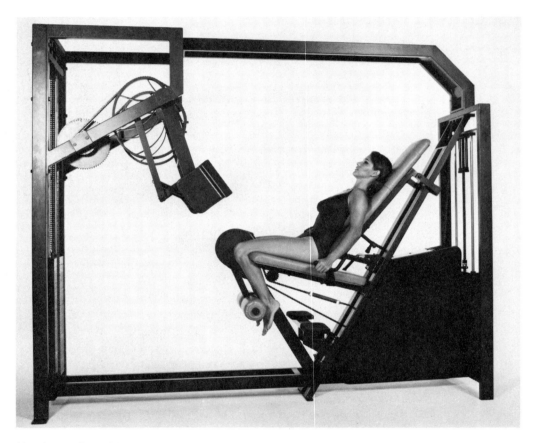

Muscles used: quadriceps
Points to emphasize:
1. Sit in machine.
2. Place feet behind roller pads, with knees snug against seat.
3. Adjust seat back to comfortable position.
4. Fasten seat belt across hips.
5. Keep head and shoulders against seat back.
6. Grasp handles lightly.

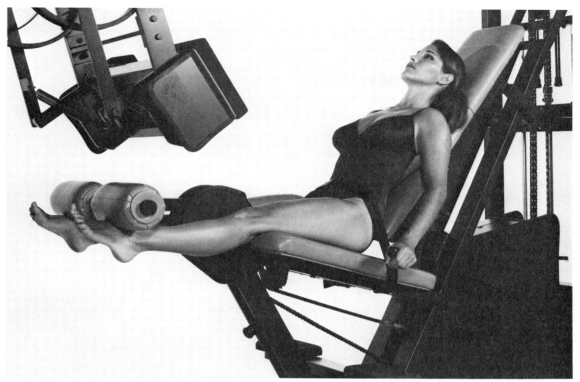

7. Straighten both legs smoothly.
8. Pause.

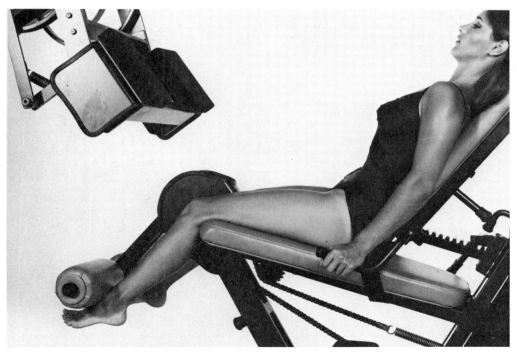

9. Lower resistance slowly and repeat.
10. Move quickly to leg press after final repetition.

Compound Leg Machine, Leg Press

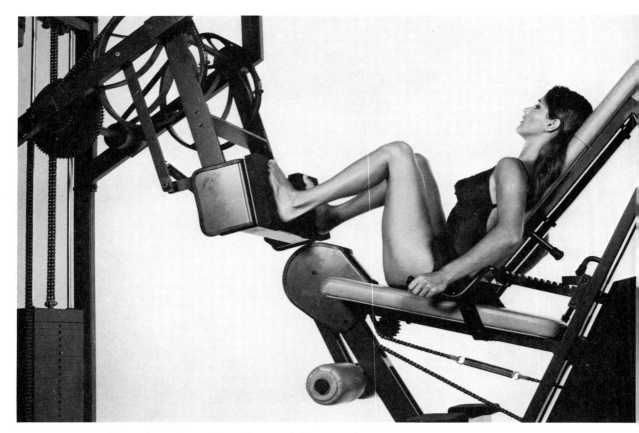

Muscles used: quadriceps, hamstrings, and gluteus maximus
Points to emphasize:
1. Sit erect and pull seat back forward.
2. Flip down foot pads.
3. Place both feet on pads with toes pointed slightly inward.

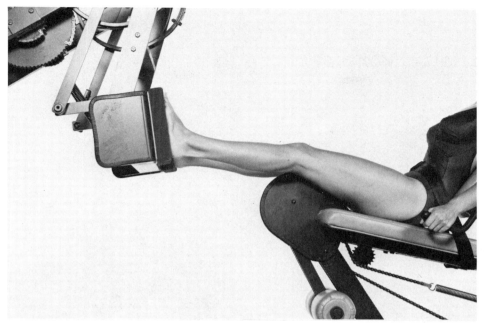

4. Straighten both legs in a controlled manner.
5. Avoid gripping handles tightly and do not grit teeth or tense neck or face muscles.

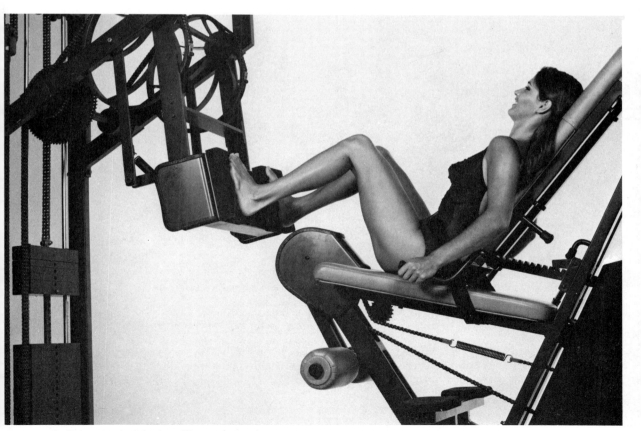

6. Return to stretched position and repeat.

Duo Squat Machine

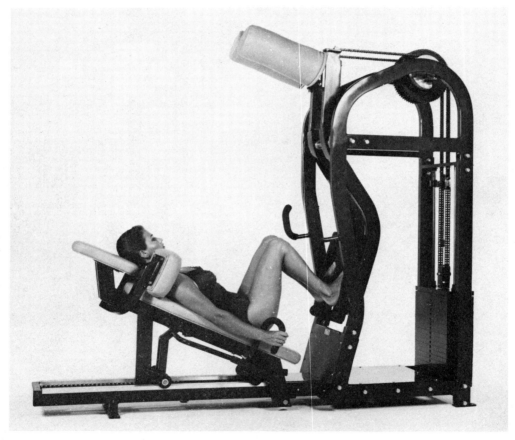

Muscles used: gluteus maximus, quadriceps, hamstrings, and gastroc-soleus group

Points to emphasize:

1. Sit on lower portion of seat. Shoulders should be under pads.
2. Place both feet at the same time on movement arms. Heels should be on bottom of foot pedals.
3. Pull up on lower right handle to adjust seat carriage. Seat is in proper position when these three factors occur as both legs straighten: (a) Negative cam fully unwinds, (b) Movement arms touch cross bar, and (c) Legs can barely lock out.

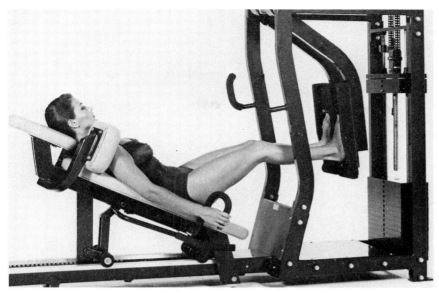

4. Straighten both legs. Keep head and shoulders on pads and hands on upper handles.

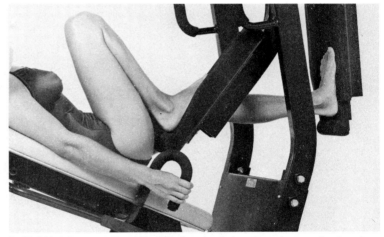

5. Hold left leg straight while right leg slowly bends and comes back as far as possible.
6. Push out smoothly with right leg until straight.

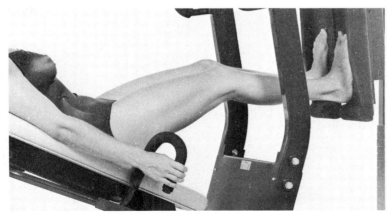

7. Hold right leg straight and bend left leg.
8. Push out smoothly with left leg until straight.
9. Alternate between right and left legs until fatigued.

Leg Curl Machine

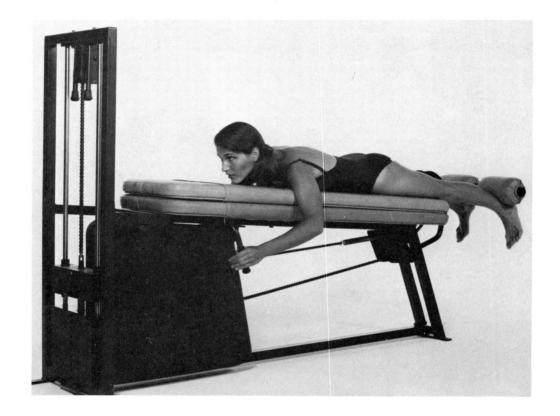

Muscle used: hamstrings

Points to emphasize:

1. Lie face down on machine.
2. Place feet under roller pads with knees just over edge of bench. Some women may require an extra pad under their thighs to put knees in proper alignment with axis.
3. Grasp handles to keep body from moving.

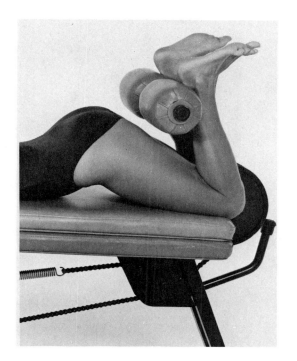

4. Curl legs and try to touch heels to buttocks.
5. Lift hips to increase range of movement.
6. Pause at point of full muscular contraction.

7. Lower resistance slowly and repeat.

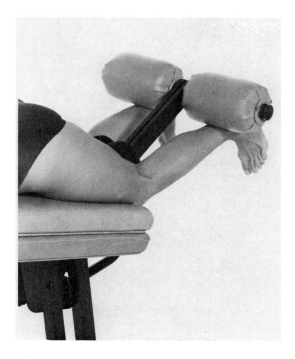

Side Leg Curl Machine

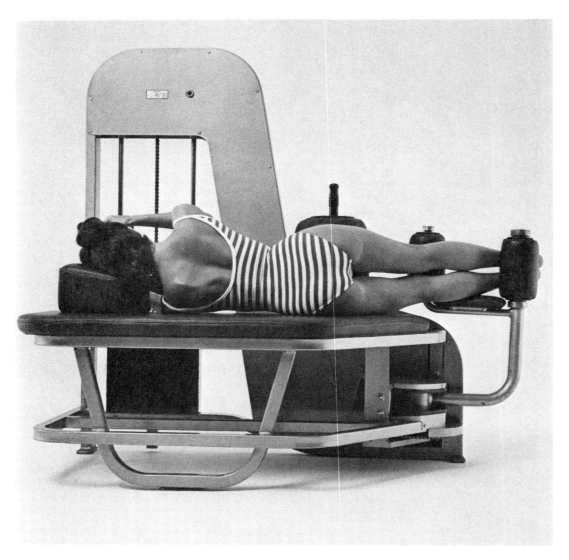

Muscles used: hamstrings

Points to emphasize:

1. Lie on left side, facing weight stack.
2. Slide lower legs between small roller pads. One pad should be on shins; the other on backs of ankles.
3. Adjust large roller pad firmly against thighs.
4. Place head in comfortable position on pad.
5. Grasp handles lightly.

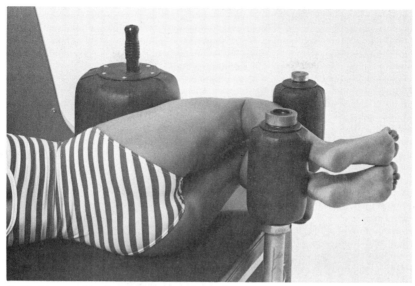

6. Curl legs and try to touch heels to buttocks.
7. Pause in contracted position.

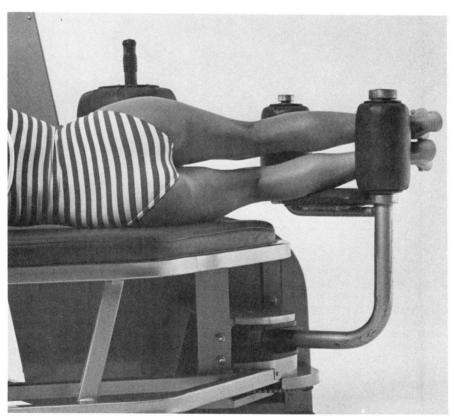

8. Lower slowly.
9. Repeat.

Hip Adduction Machine

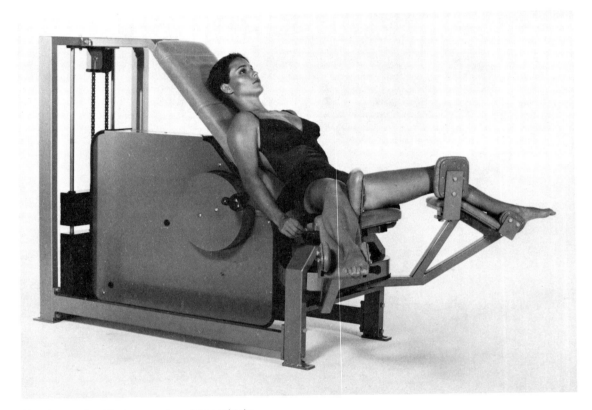

Muscles used: adductor muscles of inner thighs
Points to emphasize:
1. Adjust lever on right side of machine for range of movement.
2. Sit in machine and place knees and ankles on movement arm in a spread-legged position. The inner thighs and knees should be firmly against the resistance pads. Some women may need an extra back pad.
3. Fasten seat belt.
4. Keep head and shoulders against seat back.

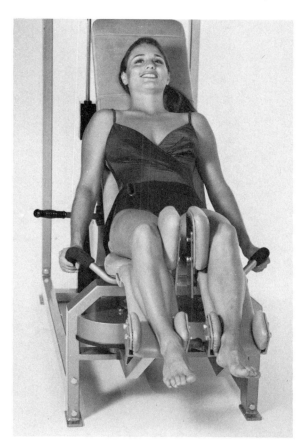

5. Pull knees and thighs smoothly together. To better isolate the adductor muscles, keep the feet pointed inward and pull with the thighs, not the lower legs.
6. Pause in knees-together position.

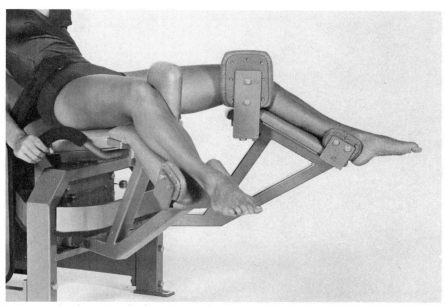

7. Return slowly to stretched position and repeat.

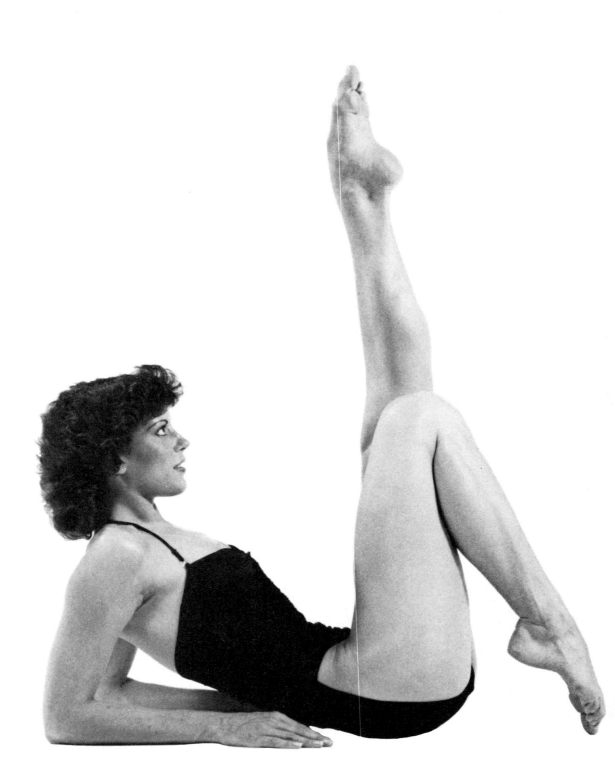

6
CALVES:
Keeping on the Toes

While wearing a skirt or a pair of shorts, stand in front of a full-length mirror. Turn your back to it and slowly rise on your toes. Notice that your lower leg muscles become pleasantly rounded. That roundness is the reason high heels will always be popular, regardless of the discomfort they cause. Curved, defined calves quite simply are beautiful.

The roundness on the back of your calves is a result of the contraction of the gastrocnemius and soleus muscles. These muscles contract when you raise your heels and stand on your toes.

On the front of your leg is the tibialis anterior muscle. Its function is to lift your toes. All three of these lower leg muscles must be correctly exercised and developed to have an attractively curved calf and a trim ankle.

Nautilus manufactures several machines that provide excellent progressive exercise for the calves. An examination of each exercise is in order.

Multi-Exercise Machine, Calf Raise

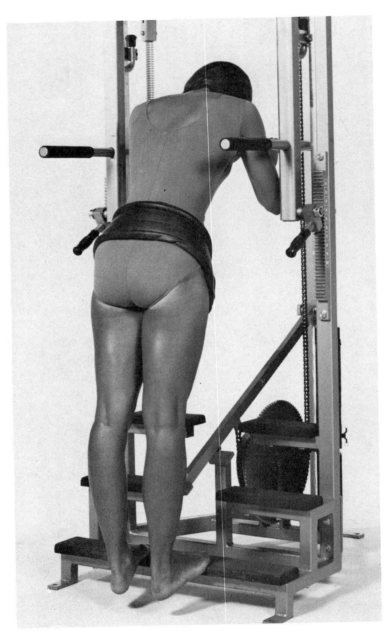

Muscle used: gastrocnemius
Points to emphasize:
1. Adjust belt comfortably around hips.
2. Place balls of feet on first step and hands on front of carriage.
3. Lock knees and keep locked throughout movement.

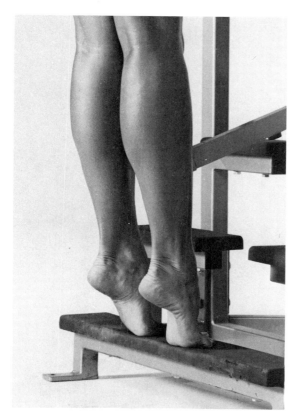

4. Elevate heels as high as possible
and try to stand on big toes.
5. Pause.

6. Lower heels slowly.
7. Stretch at bottom by lifting and
spreading toes.
8. Repeat.

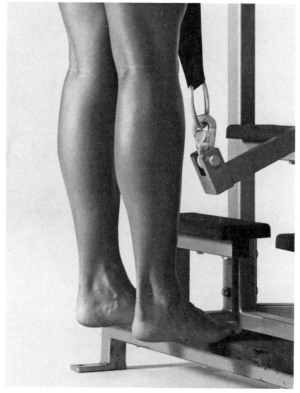

Multi-Exercise Machine, Seated Calf Raise

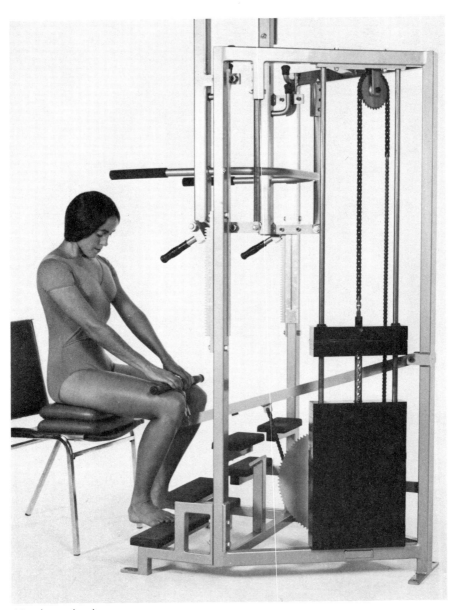

Muscle used: soleus
Points to emphasize:
1. Place chair in front of machine.
2. Attach small bar to movement arm.
3. Grasp handles and be seated.
4. Place handles on knees and balls of feet on first step. Front of seat may be raised with additional pads.

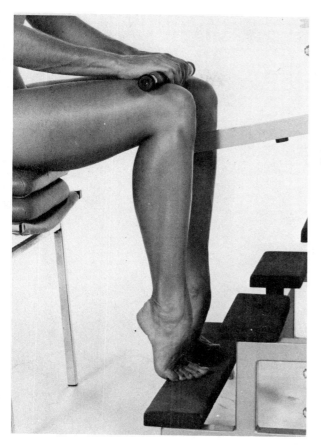

5. Elevate heels as high as possible.
6. Pause.

7. Lower heels slowly.
8. Stretch at bottom by lifting and spreading toes.
9. Repeat.

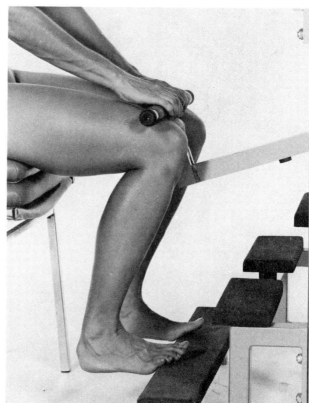

Leg Curl Machine, Foot Flexion

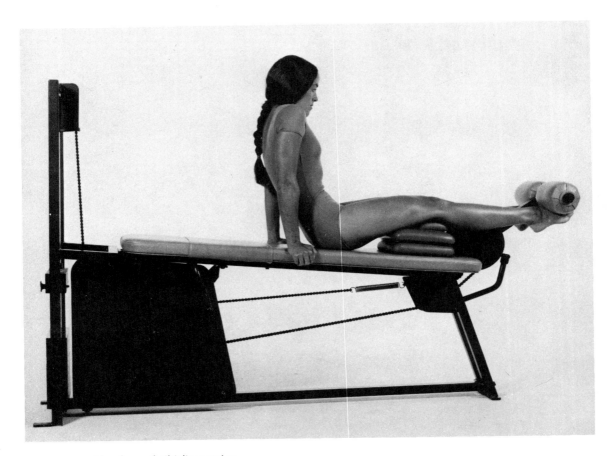

Muscle used: tibialis anterior
Points to emphasize:
1. Sit forward on leg curl machine.
2. Place toes under the roller pads and lock knees. Thighs may be elevated by putting pads under knees.

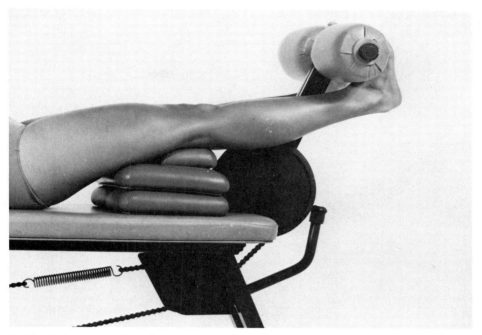

3. Flex feet against roller pads.
4. Pause in contracted position.

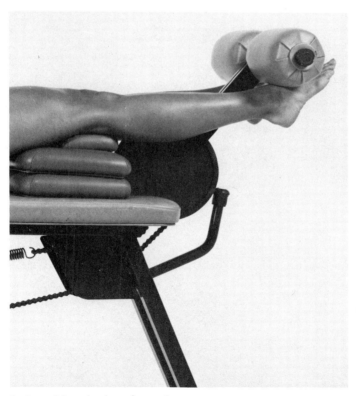

5. Extend feet slowly and repeat.

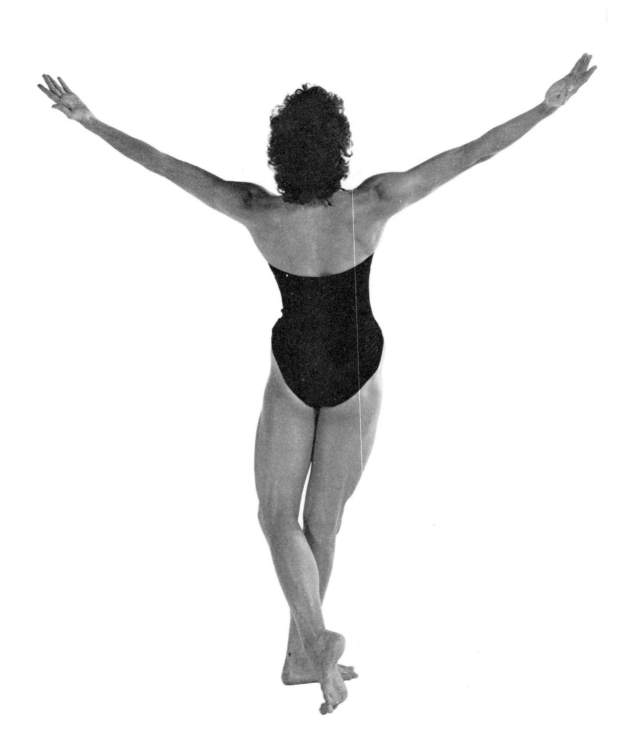

7
BACK:
Posture Plus

Is your back starving for attention? Are you taking its support for granted?

If so, read on, because a strong, straight back is not only beautiful, but it can make you look and feel healthier, more energetic, and more confident.

Good back care begins with good posture. And good posture means strong and flexible muscles, and suggests an imposing personality. The development of strong and flexible muscles also may prevent chronic back problems that most Americans inevitably suffer from.

The primary muscles of the upper back, from a posture and strength viewpoint, are the trapezius and latissimus dorsi. The trapezius is a flat, triangular muscle that extends from the base of the skull across the width of the shoulders and comes to a tapering point halfway down the spinal column. The most important of its functions is to elevate and stabilize the shoulders. A strong back guarantees confident posture, which reflects grace and allure.

On both sides of the trapezius are the latissimus dorsi muscles. They are the largest muscles of the upper body. When exercised properly, the latissimus add a pleasing "V" shape to a woman's back.

Working in conjunction with the trapezius and latissimus of the upper back are the important lower back muscles: the erector spinae. The erector spinae are composed of a large number of small paired muscles that lie on both sides of the spinal column. Extension of the spine is their major function.

The Nautilus back machines are scientifically designed to provide direct exercise for all the major muscles of this important area. Using them properly will improve your posture, shape and beautify your upper back, and provide your lower back with strong and flexible support.

Women's Pullover Machine

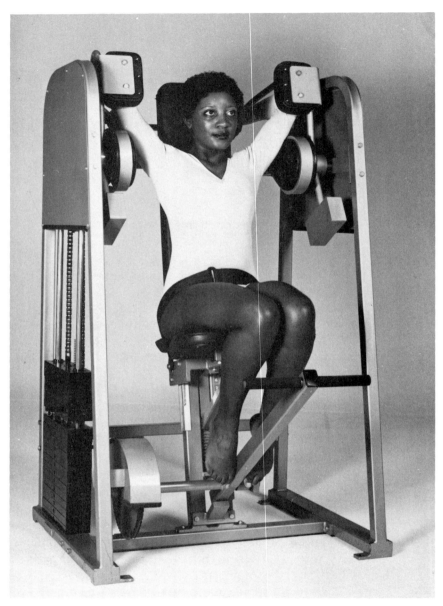

Muscles used: latissimus dorsi and pectoralis major
Points to emphasize:
1. Adjust seat so shoulder joints are in line with axes of cams.
2. Assume erect position and fasten seat belt tightly.
3. Leg press foot pedal until elbow pads are about chin level.
4. Place elbows on pads. Hands should be open and resting on curved portion of bar.
5. Remove legs from pedal and slowly rotate elbows as far back as possible.
6. Stretch.

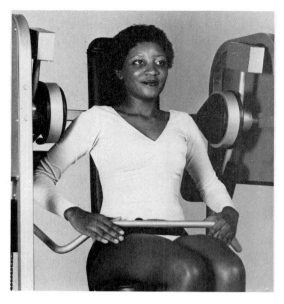

7. Rotate elbows down until bar touches midsection.
8. Pause.

9. Return slowly to stretched position and repeat.

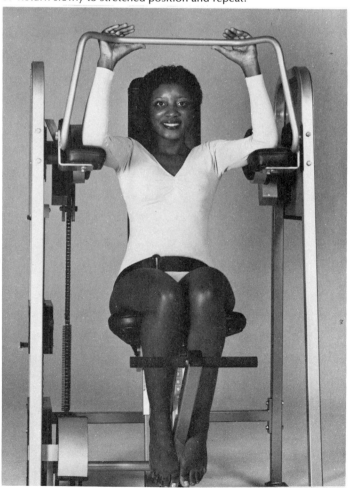

Pullover/ Torso Arm Machine, Pullover

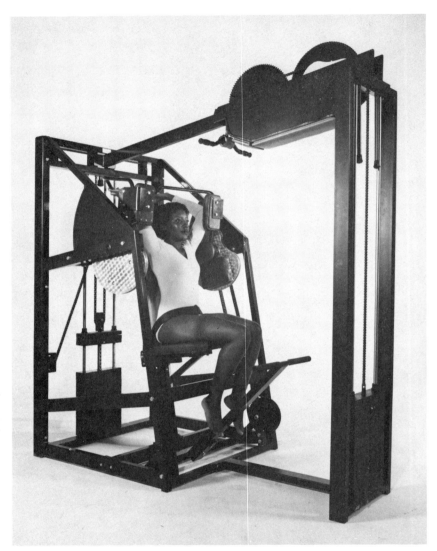

Muscles used: latissimus dorsi and pectoralis major

Points to emphasize:

1. Adjust seat so shoulder joints are in line with axes of cams. Some women may require an extra back pad to put shoulders in proper alignment.
2. Assume erect position and fasten seat belt tightly.
3. Leg press foot pedal until elbow pads are about chin level.
4. Place elbows on pads. Hands should be open and resting on curved portion of bar.
5. Remove legs from pedal and slowly rotate elbows as far back as possible.
6. Stretch.

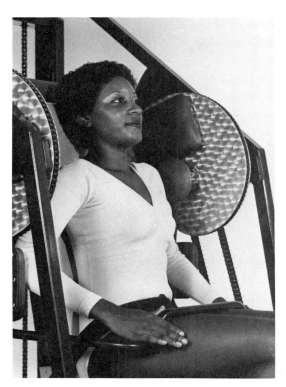

7. Rotate elbows down until bar touches midsection.
8. Pause.

9. Return slowly to stretched position and repeat. After final repetition, immediately do pulldown.

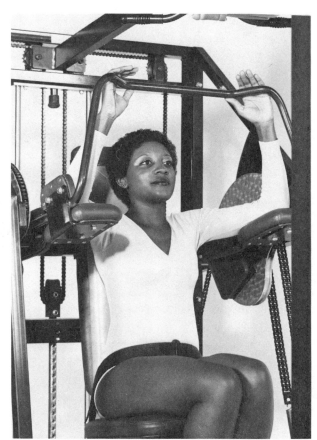

Pullover/ Torso Arm Machine, Torso Arm Pulldown

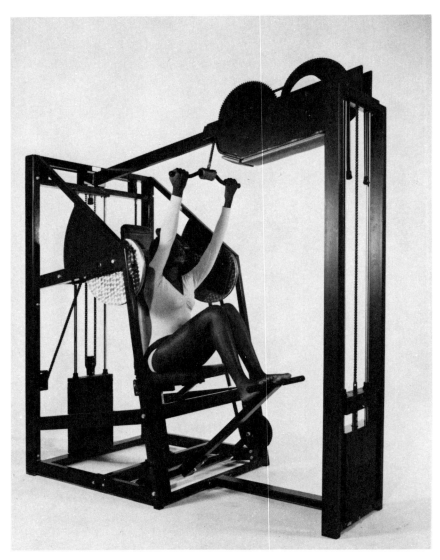

Muscles used: latissimus dorsi and biceps
Points to emphasize:
1. Lower seat for maximum stretch.
2. Grasp overhead bar with palms-up grip.
3. Keep head and shoulders against seat back.

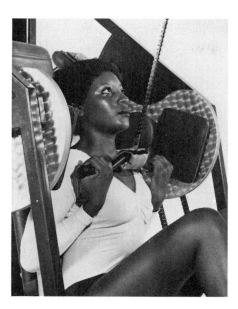

4. Pull bar to chest.
5. Pause.

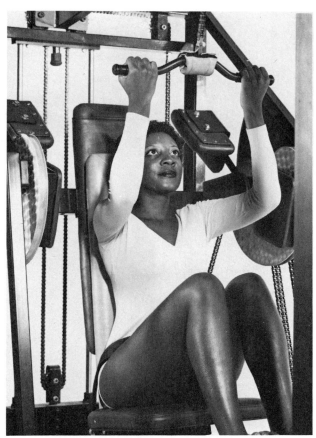

6. Return slowly to stretched position and repeat.

Behind Neck Machine

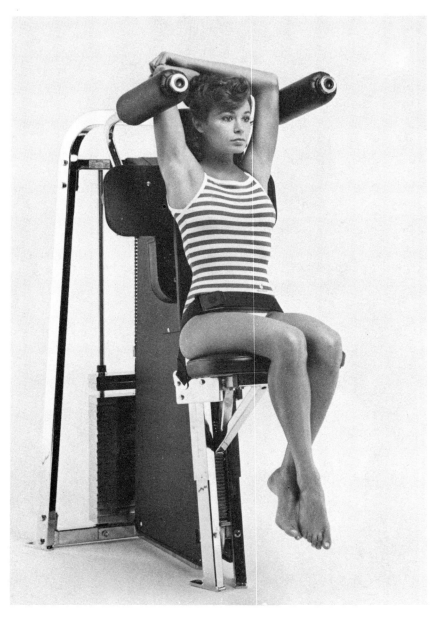

Muscles used: latissimus dorsi
Points to emphasize:
1. Adjust seat so shoulder joints are in line with axes of cams.
2. Fasten seat belt.
3. Place backs of upper arms, triceps area, between padded movement arms.
4. Cross forearms behind head.

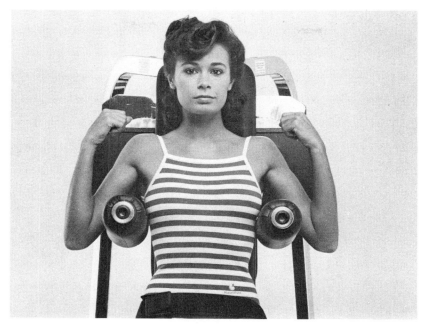

5. Move both arms downward until roller pads touch torso. Be careful not to bring arms or hands in front of body.
6. Pause.

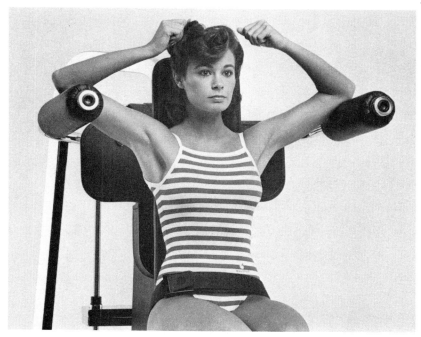

7. Return slowly to cross-armed position behind head.
8. Repeat.

Behind Neck / Torso Arm Machine, Behind Neck

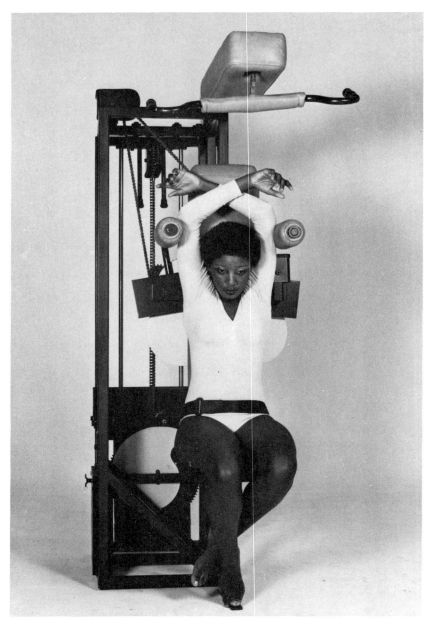

Muscles used: latissimus dorsi
Points to emphasize:
1. Adjust seat so shoulder joints are in line with axes of cams.
2. Fasten seat belt.
3. Place back of upper arms, triceps area, between padded movement arms.
4. Cross forearms behind neck.

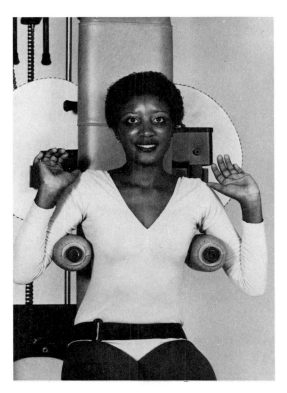

5. Move both arms downward until roller pads touch torso. Be careful not to bring arms or hands to front of body.
6. Pause.

7. Return slowly to crossed-arm position behind neck and repeat. After final repetition, immediately do behind neck pulldown.

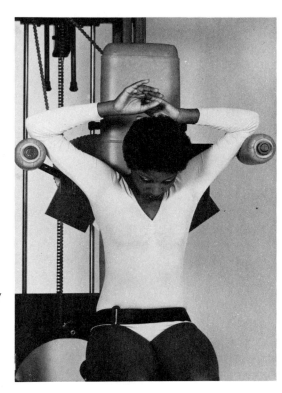

Behind Neck / Torso Arm Machine, Behind Neck Pulldown

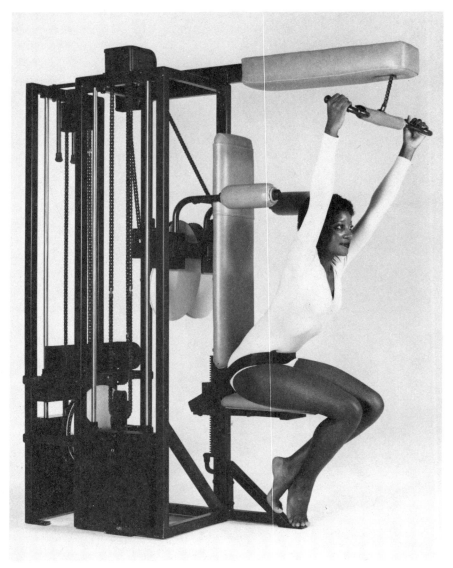

Muscles used: latissimus dorsi and biceps
Points to emphasize:
1. Lean forward and grasp overhead bar with parallel grip.

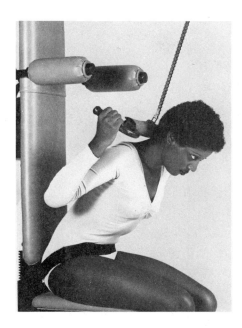

2. Pull bar behind neck, keeping
   elbows back.
3. Pause.

4. Return slowly to starting position
   and repeat.

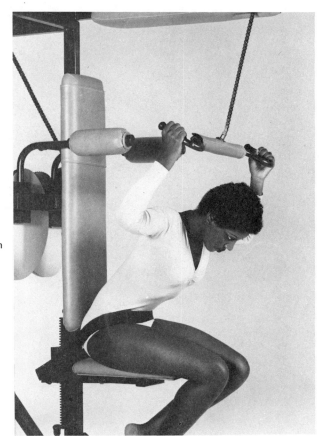

Lower Back Machine

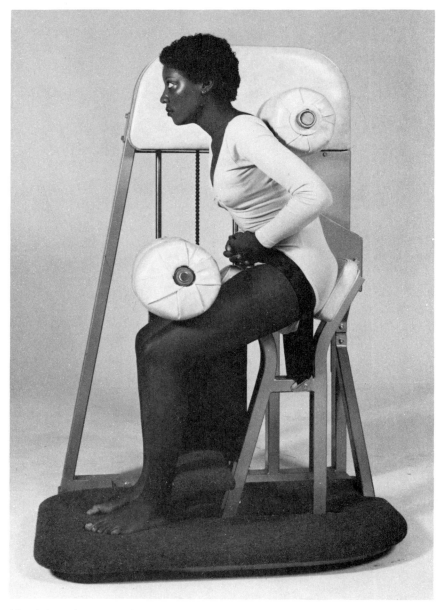

Muscles used: erector spinae group
Points to emphasize:
1. Enter machine from right side by stradding seat. Make sure back is underneath highest roller pad.
2. Stabilize lower body by moving thighs under lower roller pads. Adjust pads until thighs are secure.
3. Place feet firmly on platform or step.
4. Fasten seat belt.
5. Interlace fingers across waist.

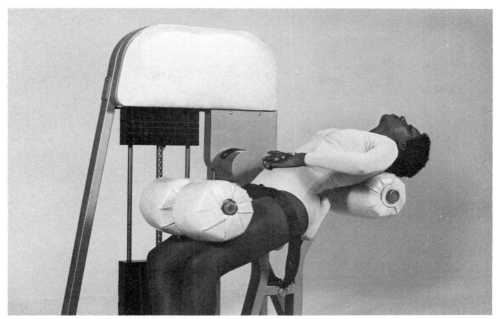

6. Move torso backward smoothly and slowly until it is in line with thighs.
7. Pause in contracted position. Do not try to arch back excessively.

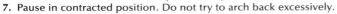

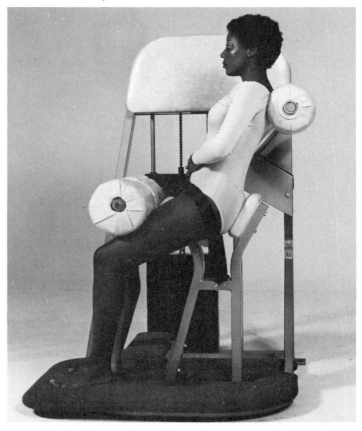

8. Return slowly to starting position and repeat.

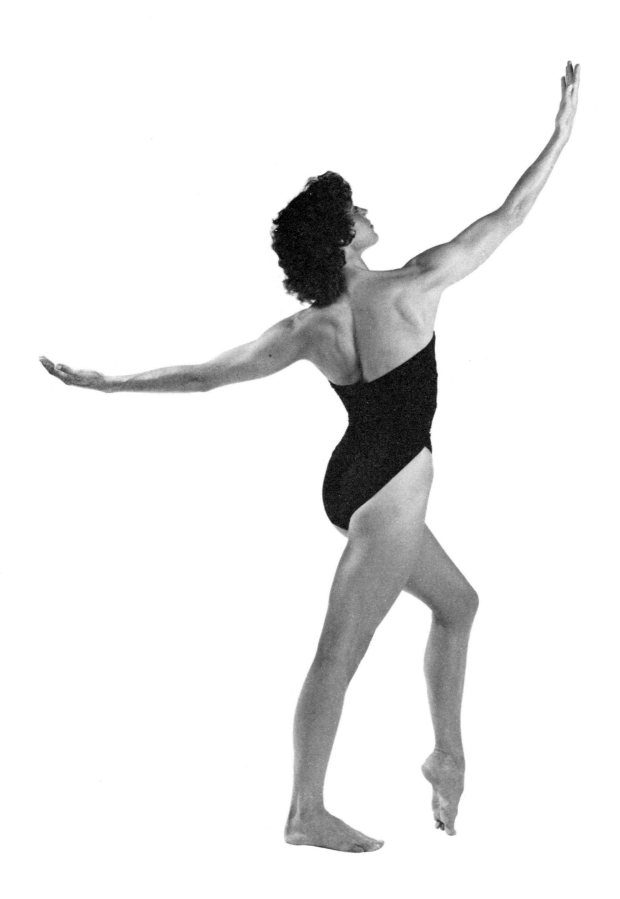

8
SHOULDERS:
Not for Men Only

What do the shoulders have to do with a shapely feminine figure? Everyone knows that it is the chest, waist, hips, and thighs that are important.

It is true that shoulders may not seem to have as much significance as well-formed breasts, a slim waist, and firm thighs. But the shoulders can be enhanced and strengthened by proper exercise on Nautilus machines. Strong shoulders will help prevent or alleviate figure problems such as slumped or rounded posture. They will tone the muscles to give you a well-conditioned, rather than a bony shoulder line. Perhaps most importantly, proper exercise will make the shoulders look broader.

Broad shoulders, you say, are masculine. Broad shoulders are masculine, but they also can be feminine.

In general, women have wider hips than men because of their hormones and genetic makeup. As compared to men, women also have narrower shoulders. The width and narrowness of these two focal points in the human body help to create an illusion. A woman, for example, who has wide hips and narrow shoulders appears to have wider hips than she actually does because of the narrowness of her shoulders.

Thus, any woman who wants her hips to appear narrower should broaden her shoulders. Broad, well-conditioned shoulders nicely balance the female tendency to wide hips.

The shoulder bones do not actually broaden. What adds width to the shoulders is the strengthening of the deltoid muscles.

The deltoid is a triangular muscle that is draped over the shoulder. One angle points down the arm and the other two are bent around the joint to the front and back. The deltoid helps to move the upper arm forward, sideways, and backward. Worked properly, the deltoid becomes rounded and shapely and contributes sex appeal and balance to the feminine body.

Broad shoulders, most definitely, are not for men only.

Lateral Raise Machine

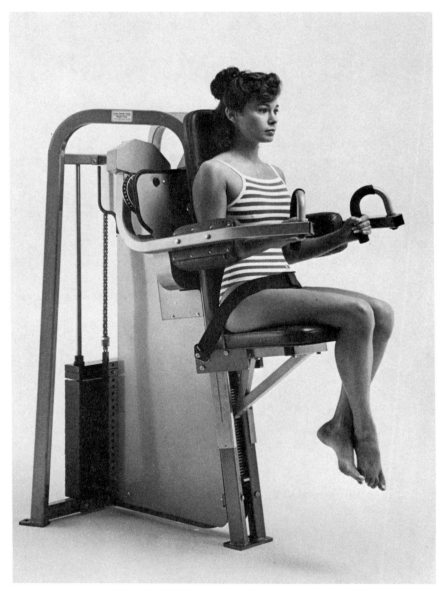

Muscle used: deltoid
Points to emphasize:
1. Adjust seat so shoulder joints are in line with axes of cams.
2. Fasten seat belt.
3. Grasp handles and pull back.
4. Make sure elbows are slightly behind torso and firmly against pads.

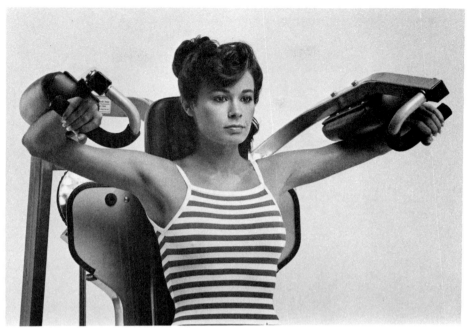

5. Raise elbows smoothly to about chin level.
6. Pause.

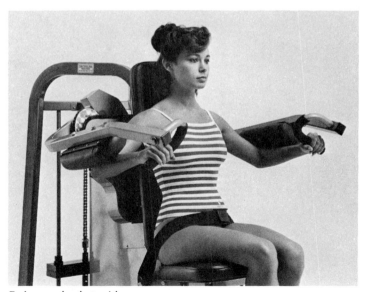

7. Lower slowly to sides.
8. Repeat.

Overhead Press Machine

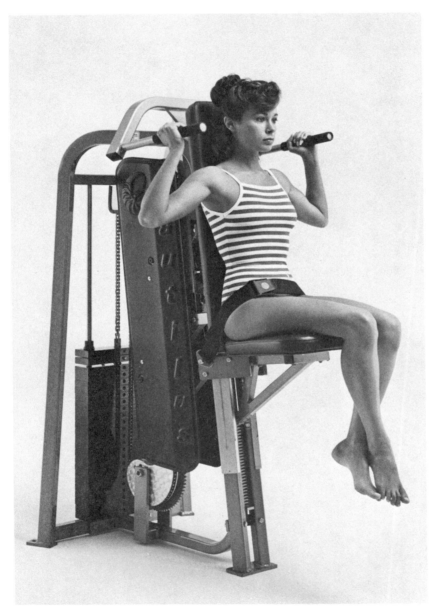

Muscles used: deltoid and triceps
Points to emphasize:
1. Raise seat for greatest range of movement.
2. Fasten seat belt.
3. Grasp handles above shoulders.

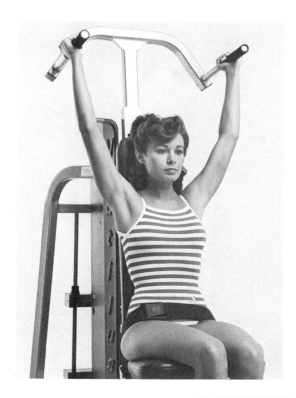

4. Press handles overhead while being careful not to arch lower back.

5. Lower resistance slowly, keeping elbows wide.
6. Repeat.

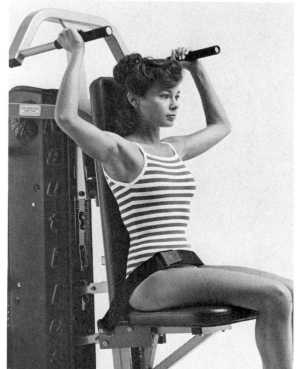

Double Shoulder Machine, Lateral Raise

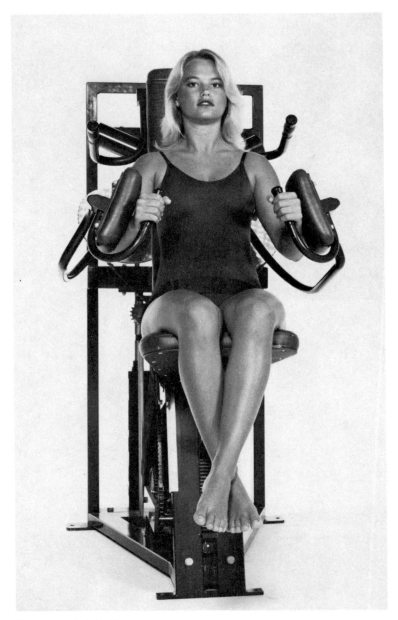

Muscle used: deltoid
Points to emphasize:
1. Adjust seat so shoulder joints are in line with axes of cams.
2. Position thighs on seat, cross ankles, and fasten seat belt.
3. Grasp handles lightly.

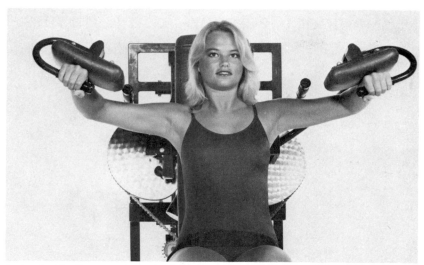

4. Lead with elbows and raise both arms until parallel with floor. Keep knuckles against pads and elbows high at all times.

5. Pause.

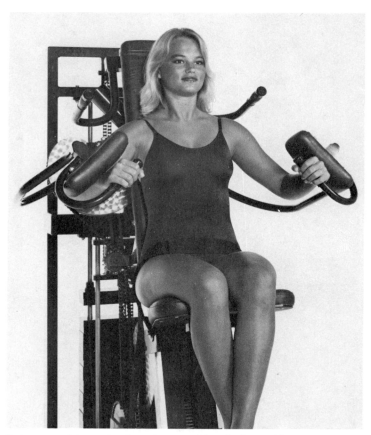

6. Lower resistance slowly and repeat. After final repetition, immediately do overhead press.

Double Shoulder Machine, Overhead Press

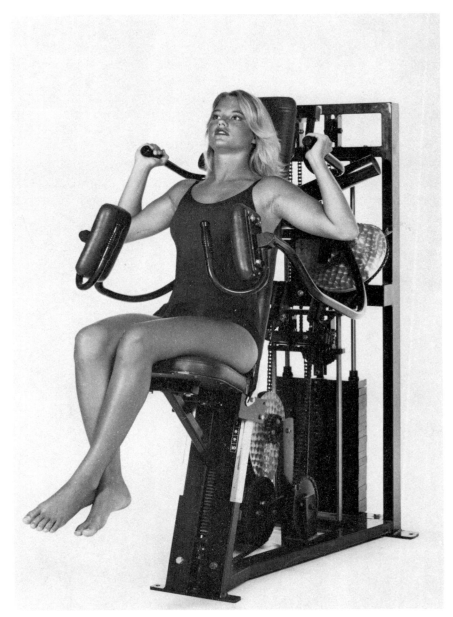

Muscles used: deltoid and triceps
Points to emphasize:
1. Raise seat quickly for greater range of movement.
2. Grasp handles above shoulders.

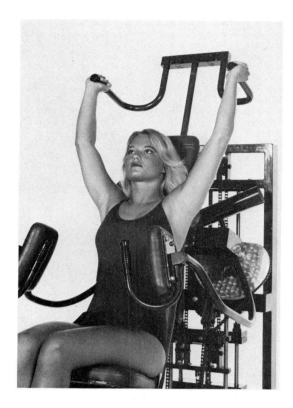

3. Press handles overhead while being careful not to arch back.

4. Lower resistance slowly keeping elbows wide, and repeat.

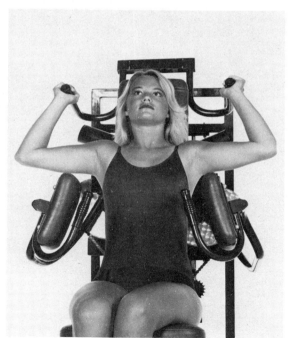

70° Shoulder Machine

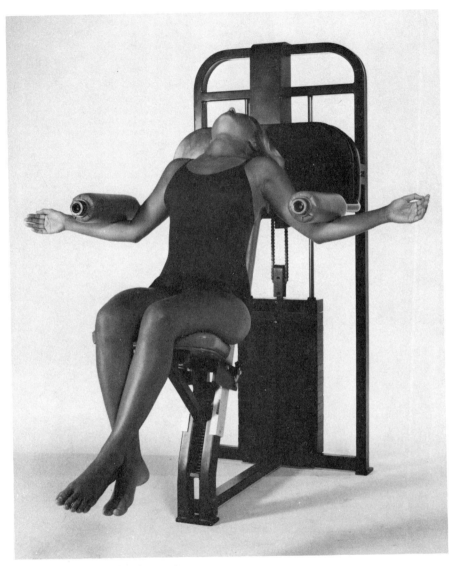

Muscles used: deltoid and trapezius

Points to emphasize:

1. Sit in machine. Adjust seat bottom so top of shoulders are in line with axes of cams.
2. Fasten seat belt.
3. Place upper arms under roller pads. Pads should be in crook of elbows or on the lower portion of biceps.
4. Extend head and rest it on pads behind shoulders. You should be looking at ceiling.

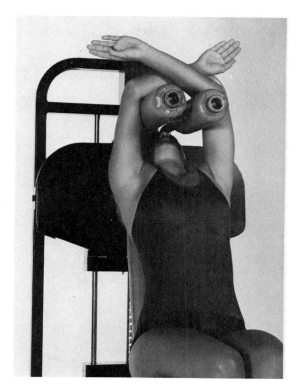

5. Move both arms in rotary fashion until roller pads almost touch over face.
6. Pause.

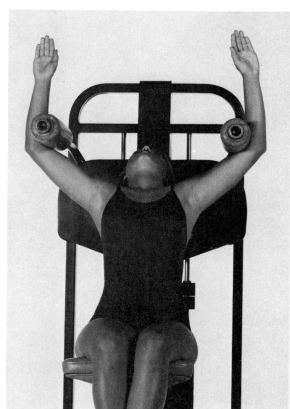

7. Lower slowly to starting position and repeat.

Rowing Torso Machine

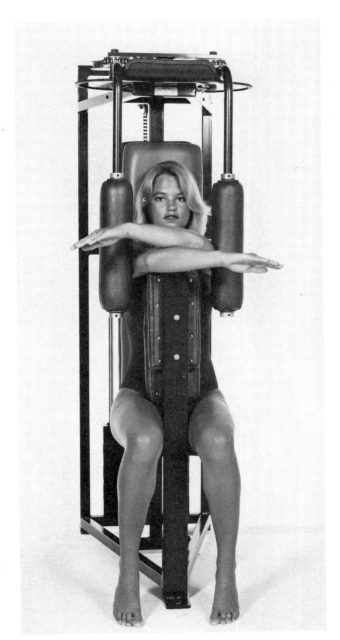

Muscles used: deltoid and trapezius
Points to emphasize:
1. Sit with back toward weight stack. Some women may need an extra back pad.
2. Place arms between pads and cross arms.

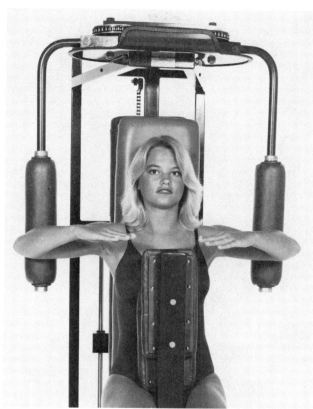

3. Bend arms in rowing fashion as far back as possible. Keep arms parallel to floor.
4. Pause.

5. Return slowly to starting position and repeat.

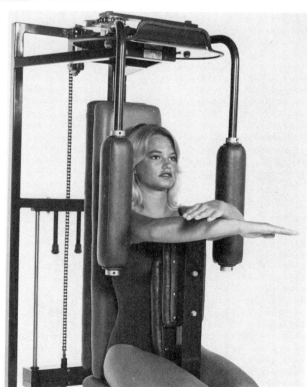

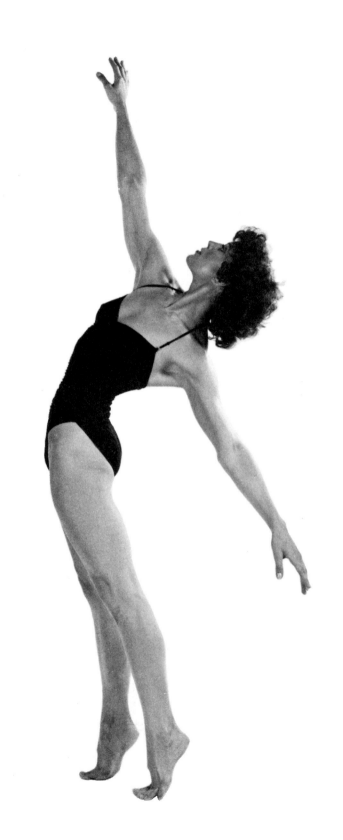

9
CHEST:
Uplifting News About Breasts

The fullness of the breasts is largely determined by genetics. That means that even before birth it is more or less settled whether the breasts will be small or large, or somewhere in between.

Although there are countless bust developers on the market that claim to add four inches or more to the bustline in a matter of weeks, medical experts agree that nothing short of cosmetic surgery can significantly enlarge the breasts. The reason for this is that breasts are composed of fat cells, milk glands, connective tissue, and blood vessels. There is no muscle in the breasts whatsoever.

But there are several muscles underneath the breasts that support and stabilize them. Support and stability also come from fibrous bands that connect the breasts to the underlying muscles. Women can do little to change the volume of their breasts, which is inherited, but the fibrous bands work in tandem with the underlying muscles, which can be strengthened and firmed. A proper exercise program will also improve overall chest expansion and torso posture, which will automatically give sagging breasts more poise. In other words, the breasts will project from a higher level on the chest and that is uplifting news!

The key muscle to strengthen and develop in your breast improvement program is the pectoralis major. Large and fan-shaped, the pectoralis major stretches across the front of your chest. When the pectoral muscles contract, they pull the upper arms down and across the torso.

Several other muscles affect your breasts, namely the pectoralis minor, subclavius, and serratus anterior. All the muscles of your chest area will become stronger and more developed as a result of disciplined Nautilus exercise.

Women's Chest Machine

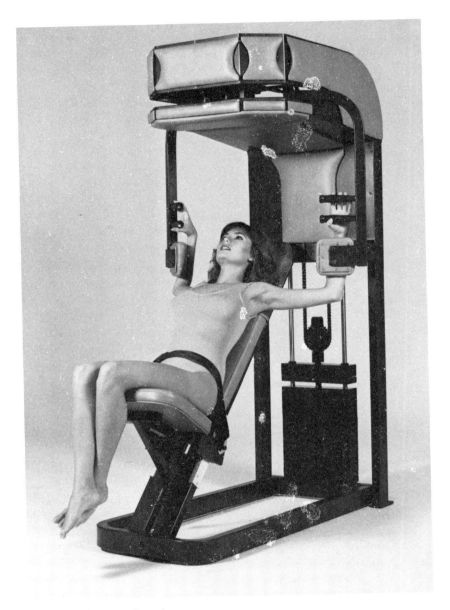

Muscle used: pectoralis major

Points to emphasize:

1. Adjust seat until shoulders, when elbows are together, are directly under axes of overhead cams.
2. Fasten seat belt.
3. Place forearms behind and firmly against movement arm pads.
4. Grasp handles lightly with thumbs around handles.
5. Keep head against seat back.

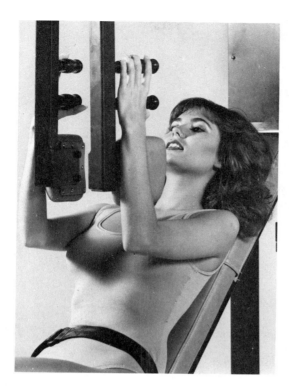

6. Push with forearms and try to touch elbows together in front of chest.
7. Pause in contracted position.

8. Lower resistance slowly and repeat.

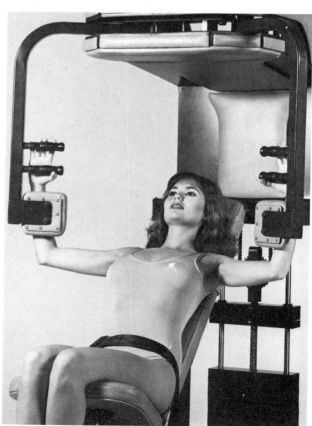

Double Chest Machine, Arm Cross

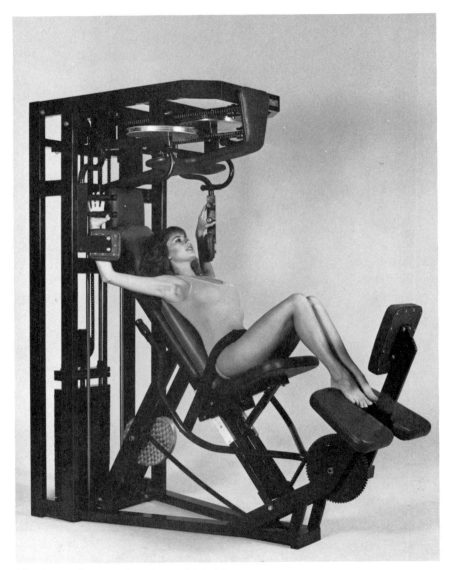

Muscles used: pectoralis major and deltoid
Points to emphasize:
1. Adjust seat until shoulders, when elbows are together, are directly under axes of overhead cams. Some women may require an extra pad to put shoulders in proper alignment.
2. Fasten seat belt.
3. Place forearms behind and firmly against movement arm pads.
4. Grasp handles lightly with thumbs around handles.
5. Keep head against seat back.

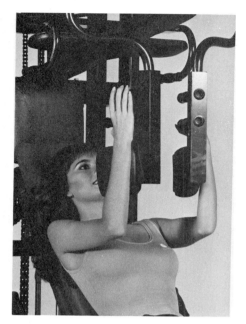

6. Push with forearms and try to touch elbows together in front of chest.
7. Pause.

8. Lower resistance slowly and repeat. After final repetition, immediately do decline press.

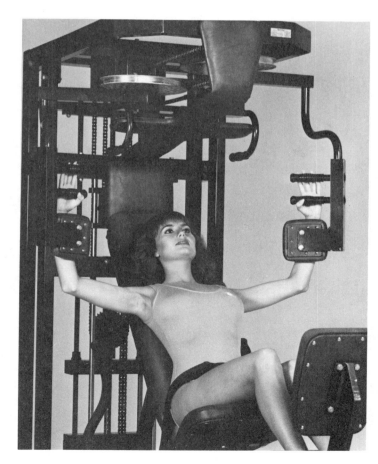

Double Chest Machine, Decline Press

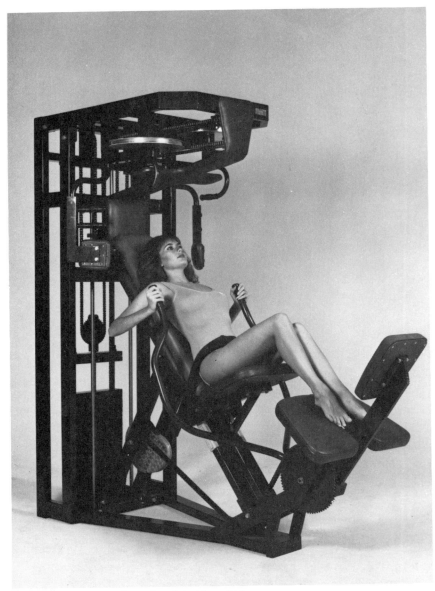

Muscles used: pectoralis major, deltoid, and triceps
Points to emphasize:
1. Use foot pedal to raise handles into starting position.
2. Grasp handles with parallel grip.
3. Keep head back and torso erect.

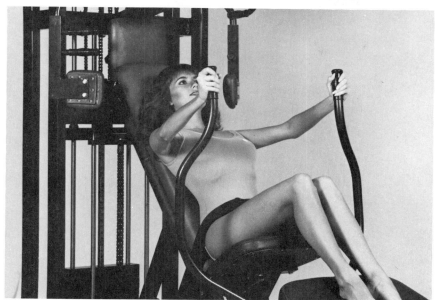

4. Press bars forward in controlled fashion.

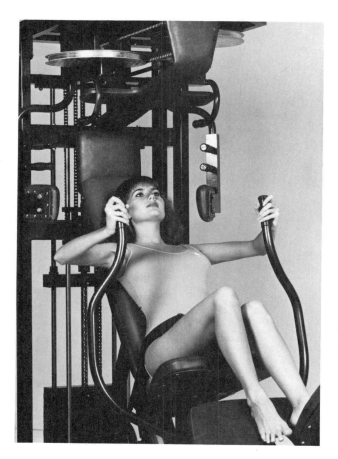

5. Lower resistance slowly keeping elbows wide.
6. Stretch in bottom position and repeat pressing movement.

Duo Decline Press

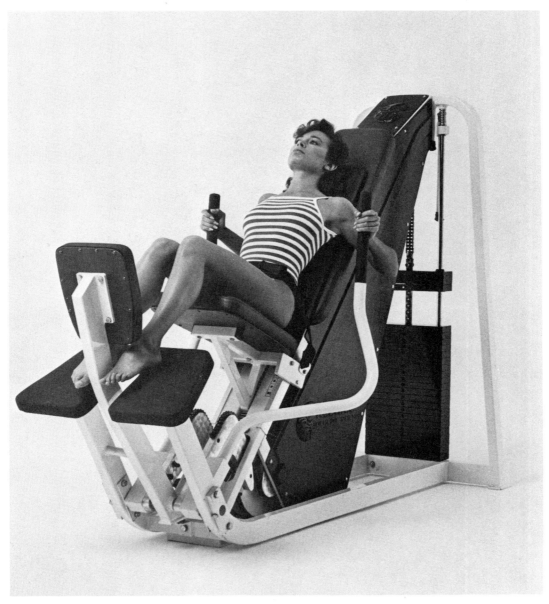

Muscles used: pectoralis major, deltoid, and triceps
Points to emphasize:
1. Use foot pedal to raise handles into starting position.
2. Grasp handles with parallel grip. You may move your hands up or down on handles and you may raise and lower seat. Both should be adjusted to allow for greatest range of movement of the involved weight stack. Some women may require an extra back pad.
3. Fasten seat belt.
4. Keep head back and torso erect.

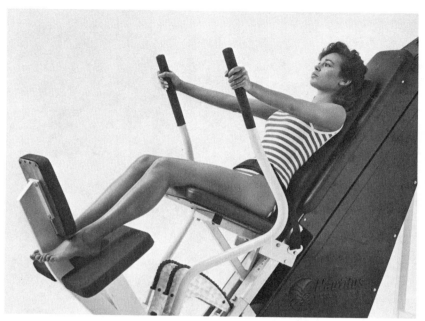

5. Press bars forward in controlled fashion.

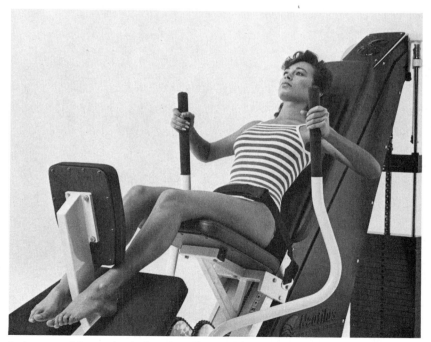

6. Lower resistance slowly, keeping elbows wide.
7. Stretch in bottom position, then continue pressing movement.
8. Repeat.
9. Movement can also be performed one arm at a time or in an alternating fashion.

10° Chest Machine

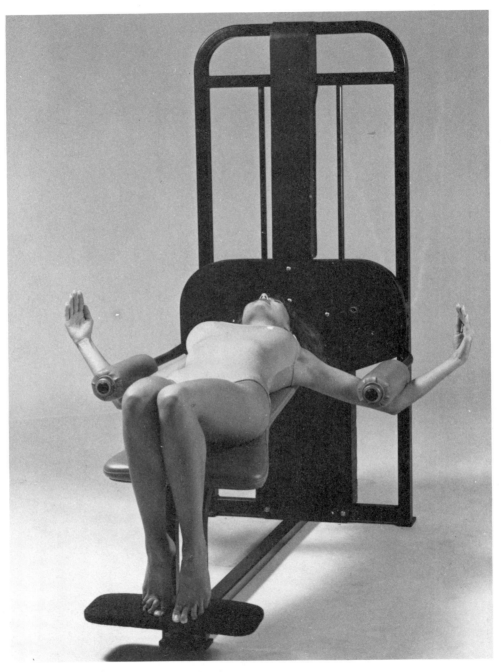

Muscles used: pectoralis major and deltoid
Points to emphasize:
1. Lie on back with head higher than hips. Adjust torso until shoudlers are in line with axes of cams.
2. Place upper arms under roller pads. Pads should be in crook of elbows or on lower portion of biceps.

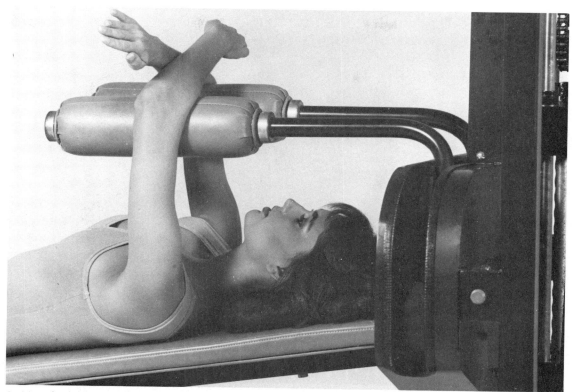

3. Move both arms in rotary fashion until roller pads almost touch over chest.
4. Pause.

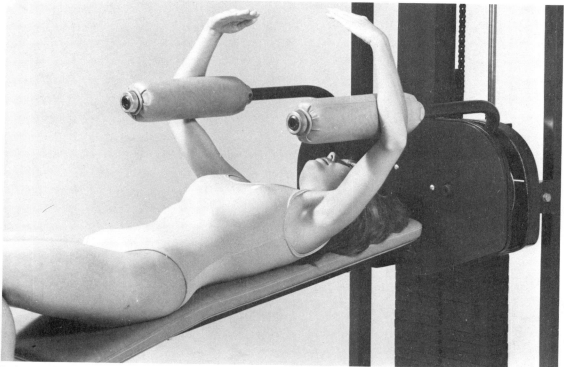

5. Lower slowly to starting position and repeat.

40° Chest/Shoulder Machine

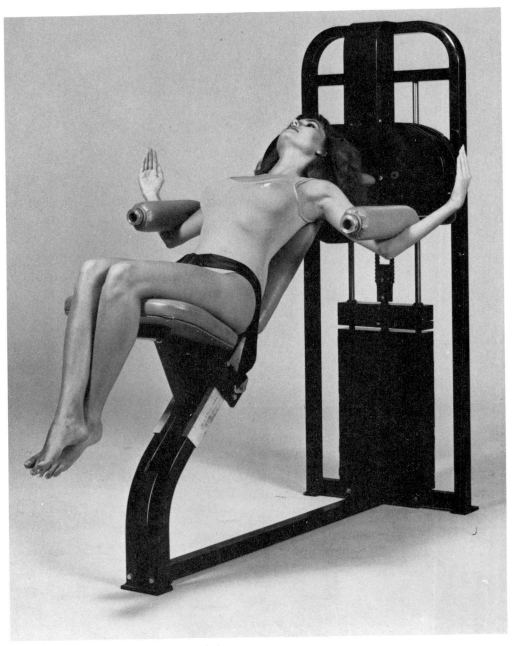

Muscles used: pectoralis major and deltoid
Points to emphasize:
1. Sit in machine. Adjust seat bottom so tops of shoulders are in line with axes of cams.
2. Fasten seat belt.
3. Place upper arms under roller pads. Pads should be in crook of elbows or on lower portion of biceps.
4. Keep head against seat back.

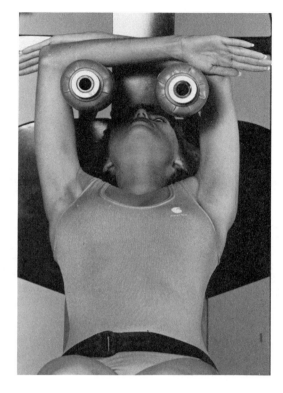

5. Move both arms in rotary fashion until roller pads almost touch over shoulders.
6. Pause.

7. Lower slowly to starting position and repeat.

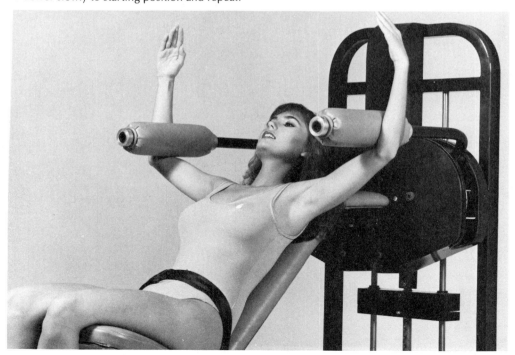

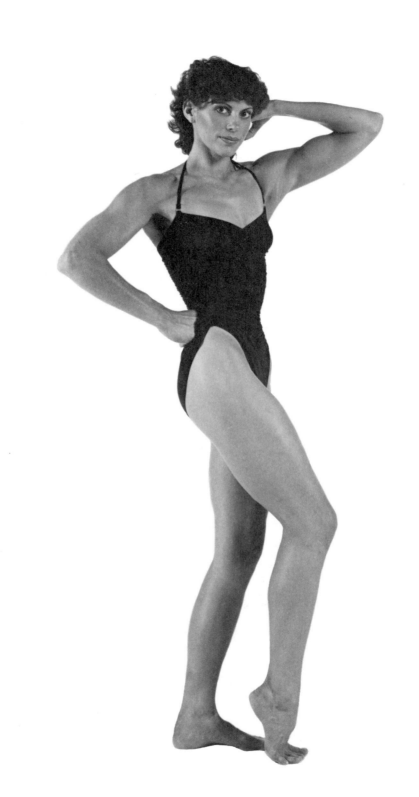

10
ARMS:
Accent on Strength

Taking a shower, getting dressed, driving an automobile, playing tennis or golf, carrying groceries, picking up and holding children, typing a letter, preparing dinner, feeding yourself, and brushing your teeth—all of these normal activities use the muscles of the arms. In fact, almost everything you do requires muscular contraction of your upper arms, forearms, and hands.

While the arms are indeed used for hundreds of daily chores, the intensity of the involvement provided them is seldom great. Few women progressively overload their arms to the extent that their muscles become significantly stronger. Yet most women have the potential to double the usable strength of their arms in six months. And will arms that are twice as strong be useful to the average American woman? Absolutely! Your performance in all activities involving the arms, both work and play, will improve. Furthermore, you will have more stamina and endurance.

Doubling the strength of your arms also improves their appearance. Much of the flabby, unattractive condition that many women have on the back of their upper arms can be prevented or eliminated. Immediately attacking the problem will decrease the chance of sagging flesh later in life. Weak wrists and bony forearms can be strengthened and conditioned also with proper training.

The major muscles of the upper arms are the biceps on the front and the triceps on the back. The biceps flexes the elbow and the triceps extends it.

The muscles of the forearms are too numerous to name. Most of them are concentrated in two masses just below the elbow joint. The mass on the outside of the forearm is formed by the bellies of the wrist extensor muscles. The inside mass of the forearms comes from the bellies of the wrist flexor muscles.

Proper exercise for the upper arms and forearms is performed on the Nautilus biceps, triceps, and multi-exercise machines. Accent these machines and watch your strength grow.

Multi-Biceps Machine

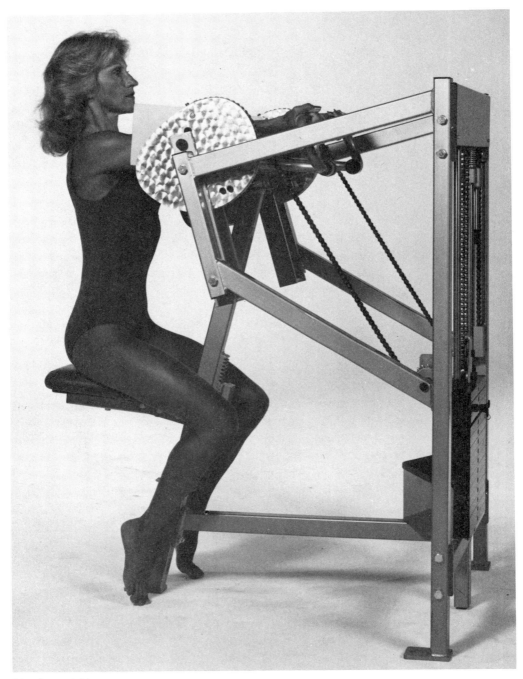

Muscle used: biceps
Points to emphasize:
1. Place elbows on pad and in line with axes of cams.
2. Adjust seat so shoulders are slightly lower than elbows.
3. Grasp handles lightly.

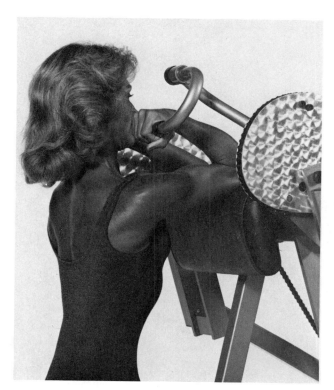

4. Curl both handles to contracted position.
5. Pause.

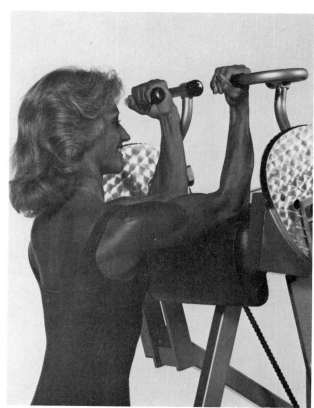

6. Lower slowly to stretched position and repeat.

Multi-Triceps Machine

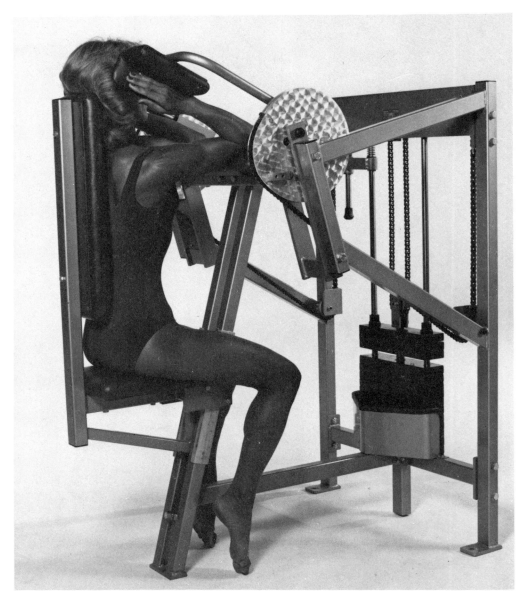

Muscle used: triceps
Points to emphasize:
1. Adjust seat so shoulders are slightly lower than elbows.
2. Place sides of hands on movement arms and elbows on pad and in line with axes of cams.

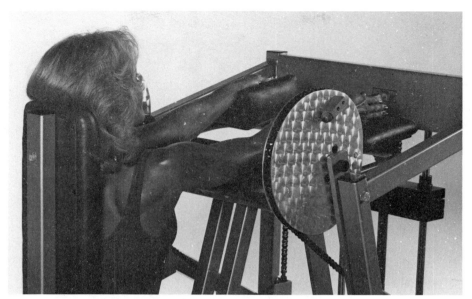

3. Straighten arms to contracted position.
4. Pause.

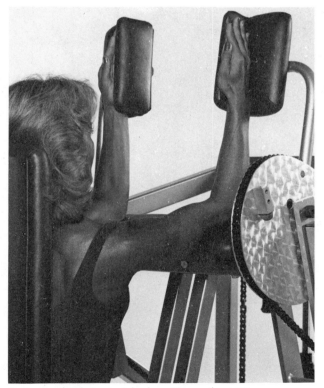

5. Lower slowly to stretched position and repeat.

Multi-Exercise Machine, Negative Chin

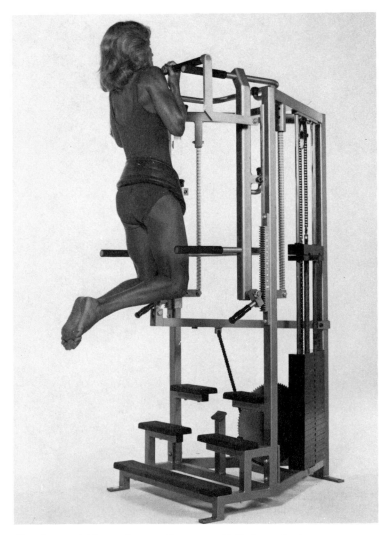

Muscles used: biceps, forearm flexors, and latissimus dorsi
Points to emphasize:
1. Move crossbar in forward position.
2. Adjust carriage to proper height. When standing on top step, chin should be barely over bar.
3. Grasp crossbar in an underhand manner with palms toward the torso.
4. Climb steps.
5. Place chin over bar and elbows by sides. Bend legs.

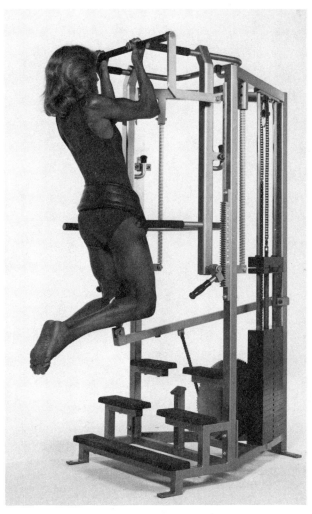

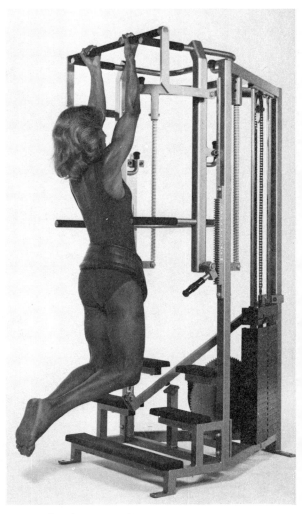

6. Lower body slowly (8–10 seconds).

7. Stretch at bottom position.
8. Climb up and repeat.

Multi-Exercise Machine, Negative Dip

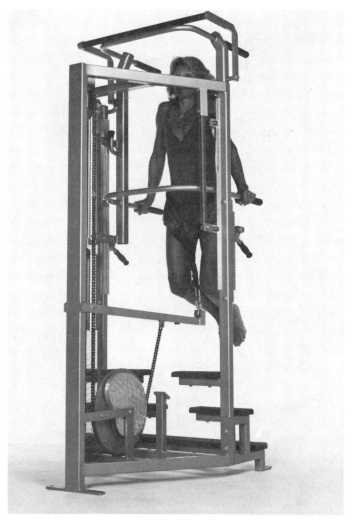

Muscles used: triceps, deltoid, and pectoralis major
Points to emphasize:
1. Adjust carriage to proper level. It is important to allow ample stretch in bottom position.
2. Climb steps.
3. Lock elbows and bend legs.

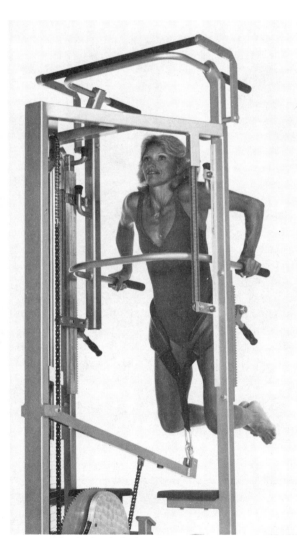

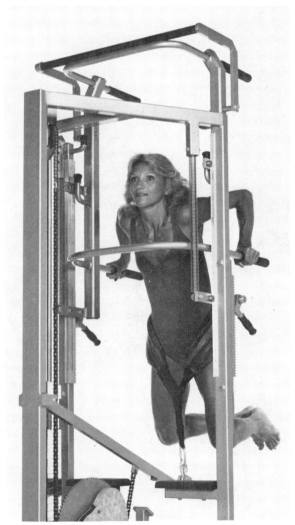

4. Lower body slowly by bending arms (8–10 seconds).

5. Stretch at bottom position.
6. Climb up and repeat.

Multi-Exercise Machine, Wrist Curl

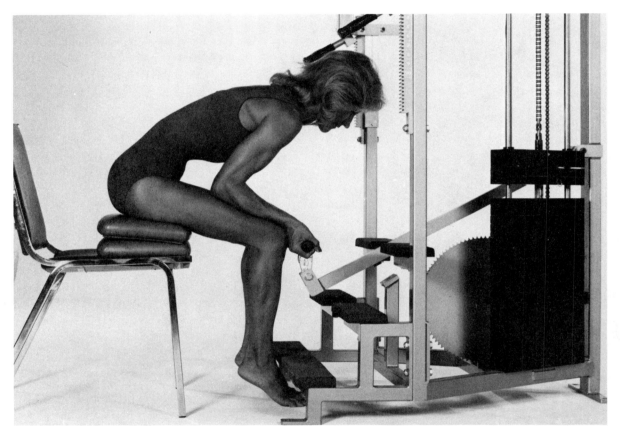

Muscles used: wrist flexor group

Points to emphasize:

1. Sit in front of machine, using small bench or chair, with toes under first step. Pad seat if necessary until hips are higher than knees.
2. Attach small bar to movement arm.
3. Grasp handles in palms-up fashion.
4. Place forearms firmly against thighs.
5. Lean forward to isolate forearm flexors. The angle between the upper arms and forearms should be less than 90 degrees.

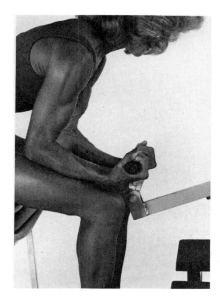

6. Curl small bar upward.
7. Pause.

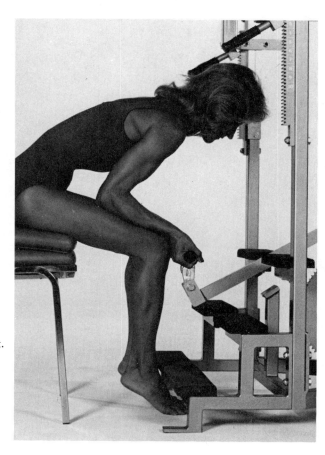

8. Lower resistance slowly and repeat.

Multi-Exercise Machine, Reverse Wrist Curl

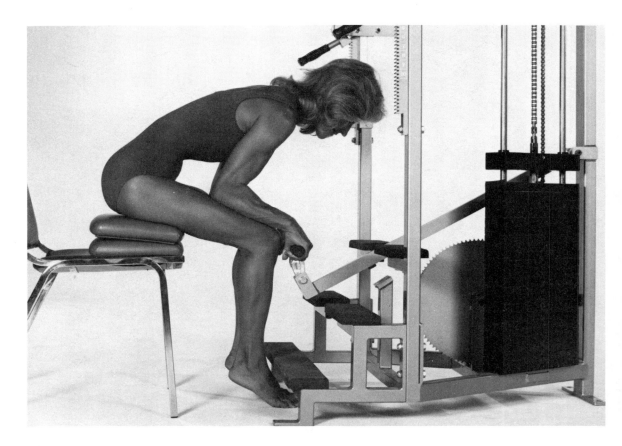

Muscles used: wrist extensor group
Points to emphasize:
1. Sit in front of machine, using small bench or chair, with toes under first step. Pad seat if necessary until hips are higher than knees.
2. Attach small handle directly to movement arm.
3. Grasp handles in palms-down fashion.
4. Place forearms firmly against thighs.

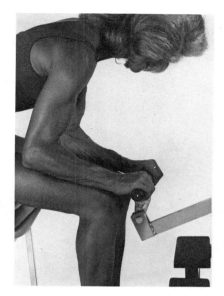

5. Reverse curl small bar upward.
6. Pause.

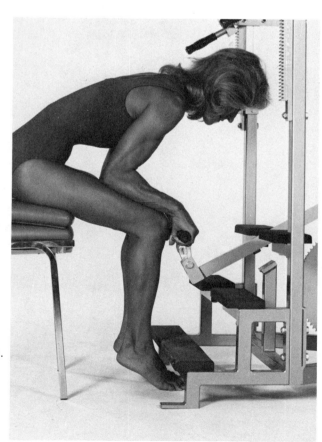

7. Lower resistance slowly and repeat.

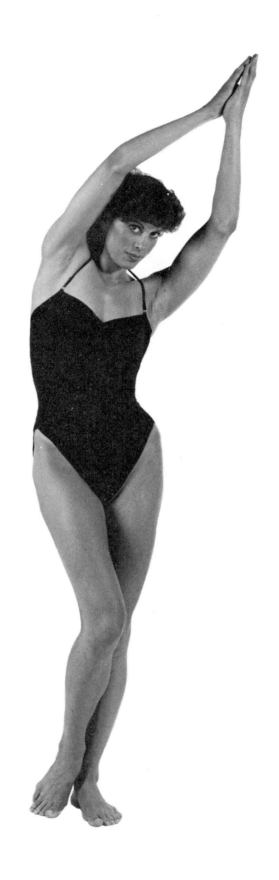

11
WAIST:
Slim and Sexy

A slim, firm waistline has sex appeal. It also keeps a woman young and athletic-looking. A midsection that is soft and thickening indicates that a woman is not in shape, and that the youthfulness of her figure is disappearing.

Keeping the muscles that gird the waist strong has other benefits as well. They support the stomach and intestines during digestion. They protect the internal organs from blows. They keep the pelvis in proper alignment. They adjust easily to the stress of pregnancy and childbirth. When neglected, these muscles provide only limited support, and every one of those benefits is impaired.

Four muscle groups contribute to the strength and contour of the midsection. The rectus abdominis muscles extend vertically from the sternum to the pubic bone. The external and internal obliques run on an angle from the ribs to the hips. The transverse muscles cross horizontally under the other three groups. All four muscle groups work together to form a natural girdle around the waist.

The most efficient way to strengthen and condition this natural girdle of muscle is by correct use of the Nautilus abdominal and rotary torso machines. You will begin to notice results from these two machines in a matter of weeks. In a moderate time, your waist will become slimmer and firmer. You will notice improvement in your pride and self-image as well.

"But will my sex appeal improve?" you ask.

Don't worry. When your waist gets slim and firm, you will not need to ask.

Abdominal Machine (Old)

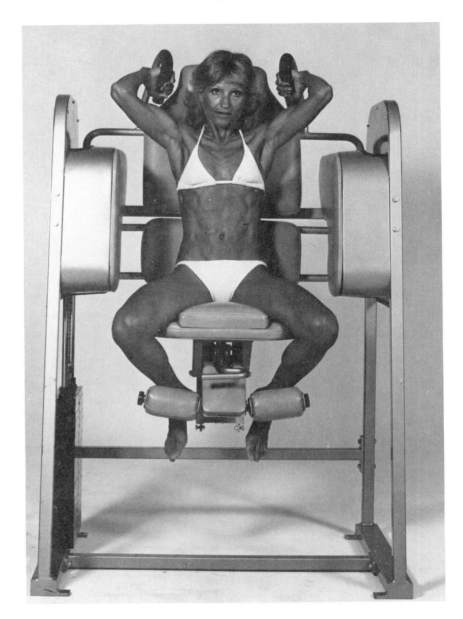

Muscle used: rectus abdominis

Points to emphasize:

1. Sit in machine.
2. Locate axis of rotation on right side.
3. Adjust seat so axis of rotation is at same level as lower ribs.
4. Place ankles behind roller pads.
5. Spread knees and sit erect.
6. Grasp handles.
7. Keep shoulders and head firmly against seat back.

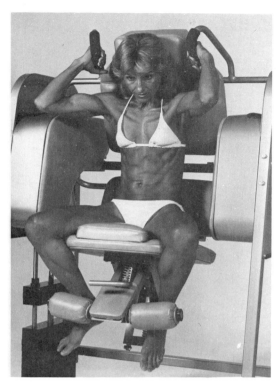

8. Shorten the distance between rib cage and navel by contracting abdominals only. Do not pull with latissimus or triceps muscles.
9. Keep legs relaxed and knees wide as seat bottom is elevated.
10. Pause in contracted position.

11. Return slowly to starting position and repeat.

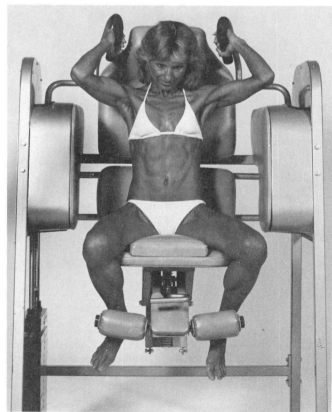

Abdominal Machine (New)

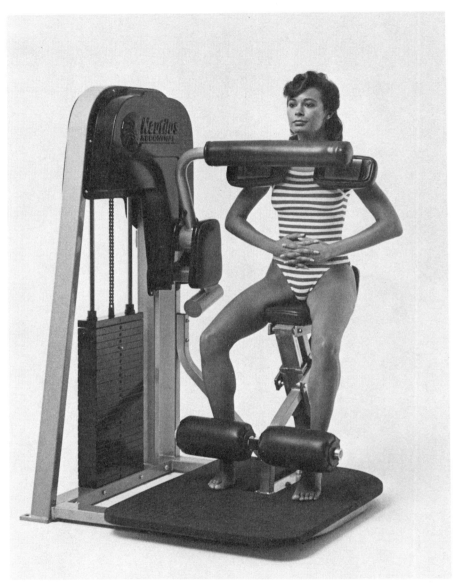

Muscles used: rectus abdominis and iliopsoas
Points to emphasize:
1. Sit in machine with swivel pads in front of chest.
2. Adjust seat until axis of rotation of movement arm is parallel to navel.
3. Hook both feet under bottom roller pads.
4. Adjust swivel pads on chest to comfortable position.
5. Place hands across waist.
6. Keep knees wide.

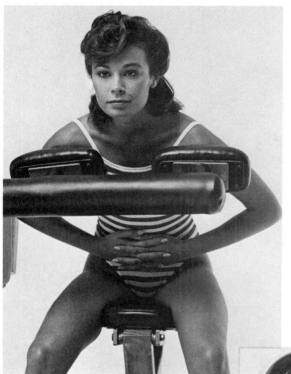

7. Crunch torso downward toward seat bottom.
8. Pause in contracted position.

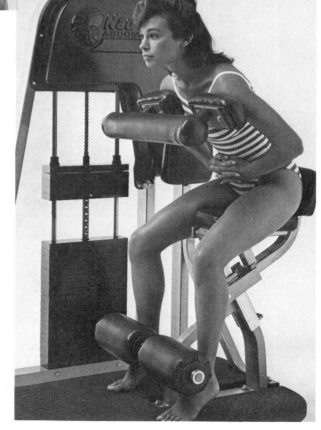

9. Return slowly to starting position.
10. Repeat.

Rotary Torso Machine

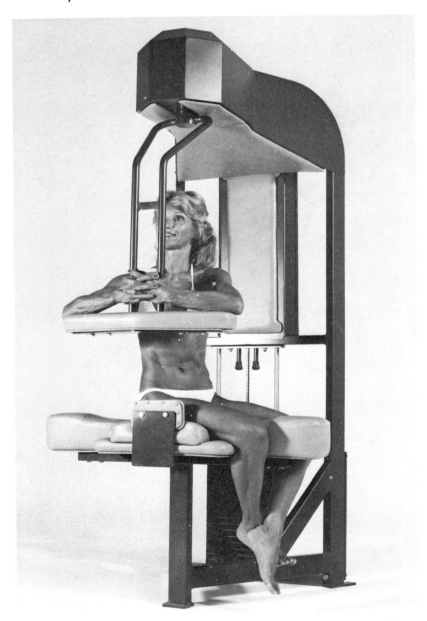

Muscles used: external oblique, internal oblique, erector spinae group, and deep posterior spinal group

Points to emphasize:

1. Face machine while standing. Weight stack should be in back and double-sided seat in front.
2. Straddle seat on right side and cross ankles securely. Do not allow hips and legs to move with torso.
3. Turn to right and place forearms on sides of pads. Right palm should be firmly against middle bar of movement arm.

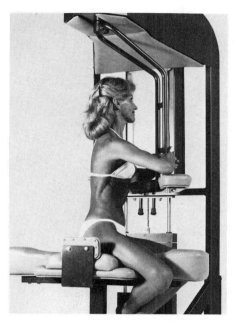

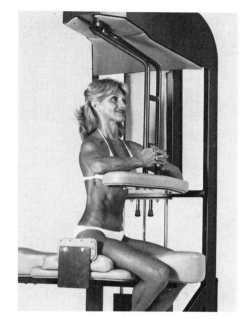

4. Rotate torso from right to left by pushing with the right palm. Do not use triceps or biceps to push or pull the movement arm. Use the torso rotators.
5. Move head with torso by focusing between parallel bars of movement arm.
6. Pause in contracted position. Rotation of torso will be less than 180 degrees.

7. Return slowly to starting position and repeat.

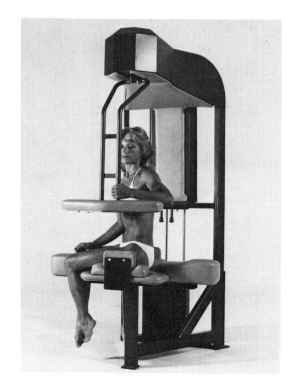

8. Straddle seat on left side of machine and reverse procedure for left-to-right torso rotation.

Multi-Exercise Machine, Side Bend

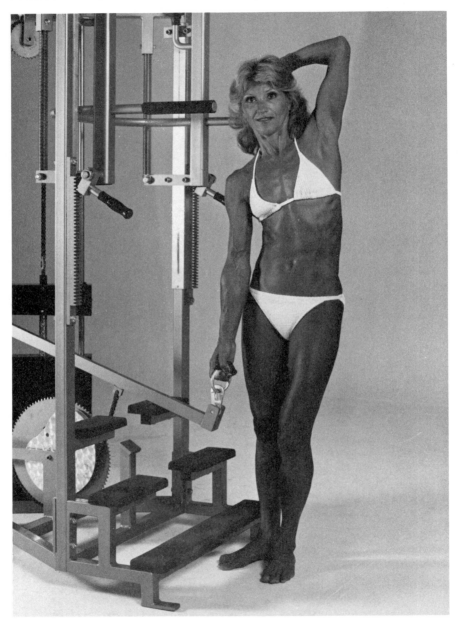

Muscles used: abdominal group
Points to emphasize:
1. Attach belt or handle to movement arms.
2. Grasp handle in right hand with right shoulder facing machine.
3. Assume a standing position.
4. Place left hand on top of head.

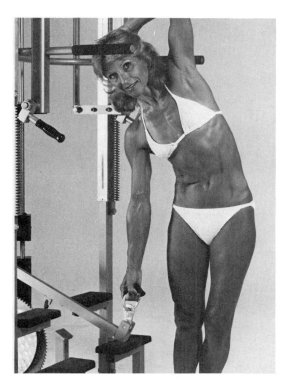

5. Bend to right side.

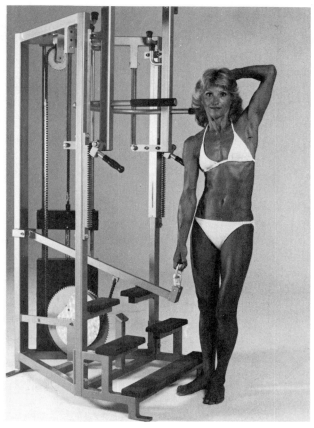

6. Return to standing position and repeat.
7. Change hands and do side bend to left side.

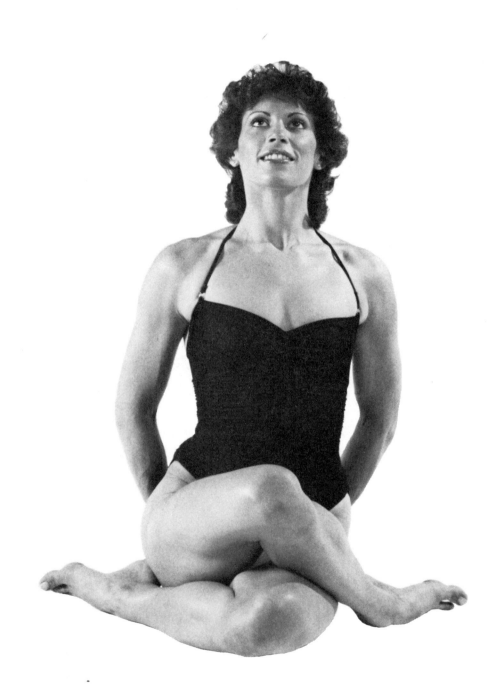

12
NECK:
The Finishing Touch

Reach up and put your hand on one of your collarbones. Run your fingers across both sides. Is there a distinct hollowness above and below these bones?

Move your hand to your neck. Squeeze lightly the frontal area. Extend your head back and feel the tissue under your jaws. Is the frontal area flaccid? Is there too much droop under your chin?

Now let your hand massage the muscles on the back of your neck. Does it feel overtense and tired?

If you answered "yes" to any of the questions above, then you could benefit from exercising your neck.

A scrawny, weak neck stands out conspiciously even in the best built woman. A strong neck is not only an addition to personal appearance, but a safeguard against injury. Whiplash and other neck injuries happen to thousands of women every week as a result of accidents. Many of these injuries would have been nonexistent if the victim's neck had been stronger. Even in simple weekend activities, there are many cases of preventable stiff necks.

At least 15 small and medium-sized muscles, the most important of which is the sternocleidomastoid, make up the bulk of the neck. To feel the sternocleidomastoid, simply place the palm of one hand on your forehead and resist as you move your head forward. Feel the side of your neck with the other hand. This muscle will stand out like a heavy cord.

The Nautilus neck machines are specifically designed to provide full-range exercise for these important neck muscles. Emphasize neck training for several months and you will not be sorry. You will be adding the finishing touch to a slim, strong, attractive body.

4-Way Neck Machine, Front Flexion

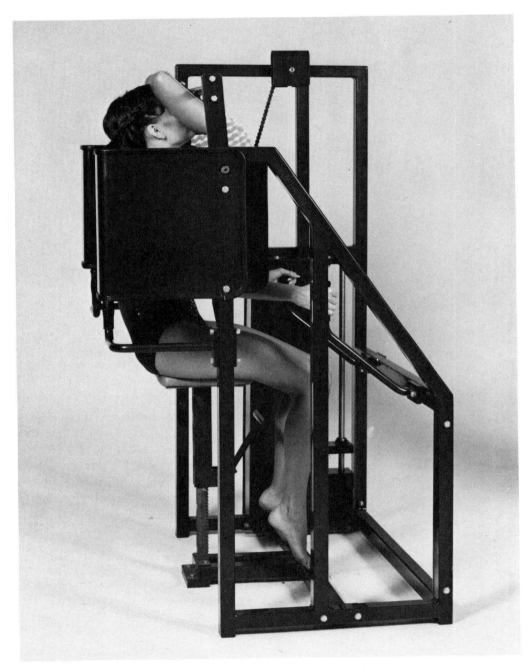

Muscles used: several on front of neck
Points to emphasize:
1. Face machine.
2. Adjust seat so nose is in center of pads.
3. Stabilize torso by lightly grasping handles.

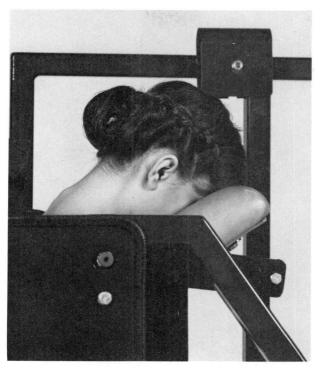

4. Move head smoothly toward chest.
5. Pause.

6. Return slowly to stretched position and repeat.

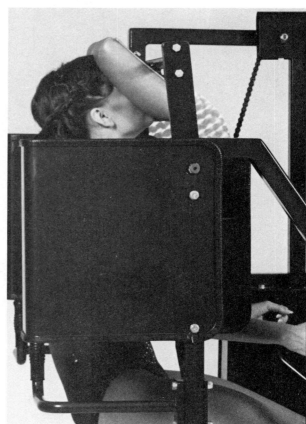

4-Way Neck Machine, Back Extension

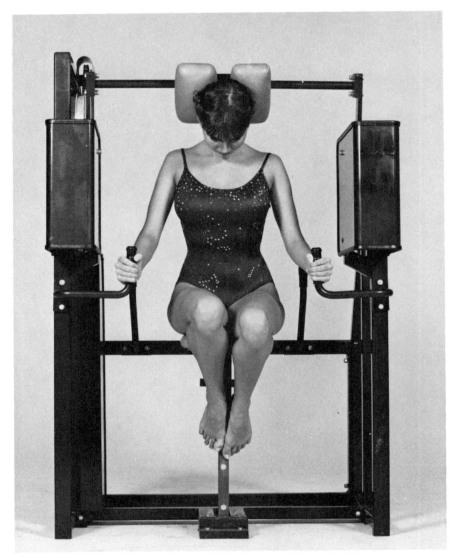

Muscles used: several on back of neck
Points to emphasize:
1. Turn body in machine until back of head contacts center of pads.
2. Stabilize torso by lightly grasping handles.

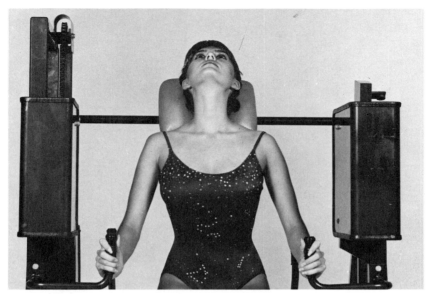

3. Extend head as far back as possible.
4. Pause.

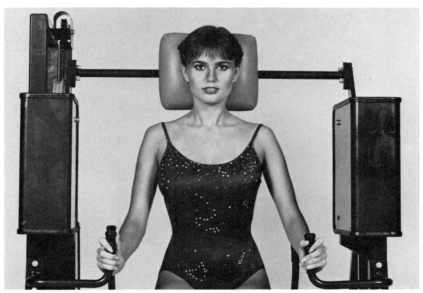

5. Return slowly to stretched position and repeat.

4-Way Neck Machine, Lateral Contraction to the Left

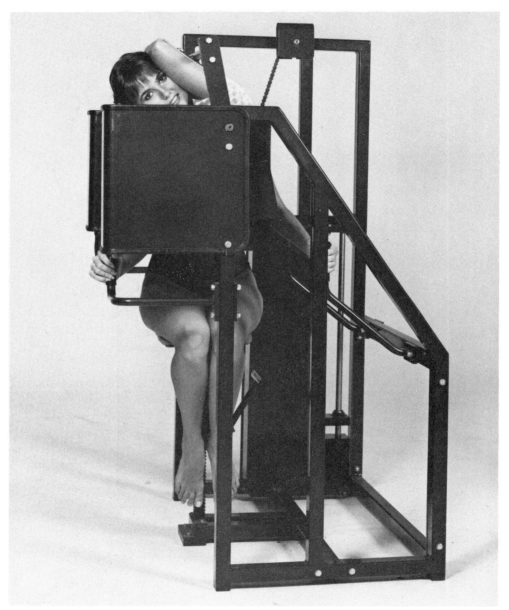

Muscles used: several on left side of neck
Points to emphasize:
1. Turn body in machine until left ear is in center of pads.
2. Stabilize torso by lightly grasping handles.

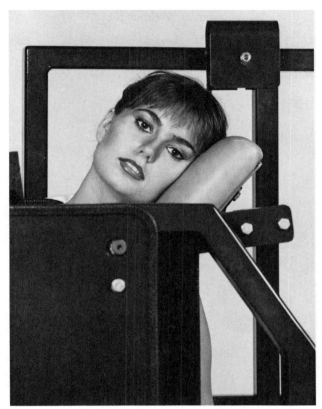

3. Move head toward left shoulder.
4. Pause.
5. Keep shoulders square.

6. Return slowly to stretched position and repeat.

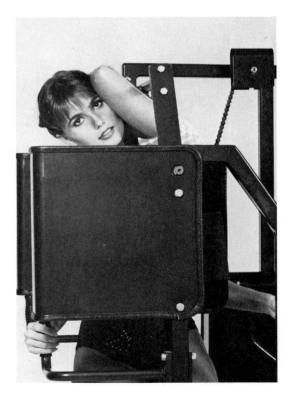

4-Way Neck Machine, Lateral Contraction to the Right

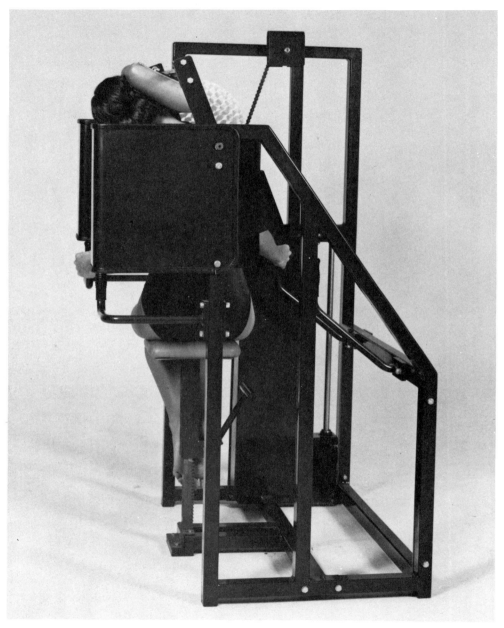

Muscles used: several on right side of neck
Points to emphasize:
1. Turn body in machine until right ear is in center of pads.
2. Stabilize torso by lightly grasping handles.

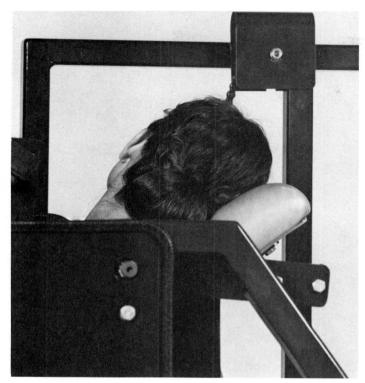

3. Move head toward right shoulder.
4. Pause.
5. Keep shoulders square.

6. Return slowly to stretched position and repeat.

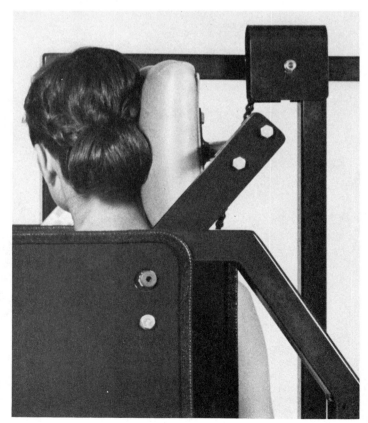

Neck and Shoulder Machine

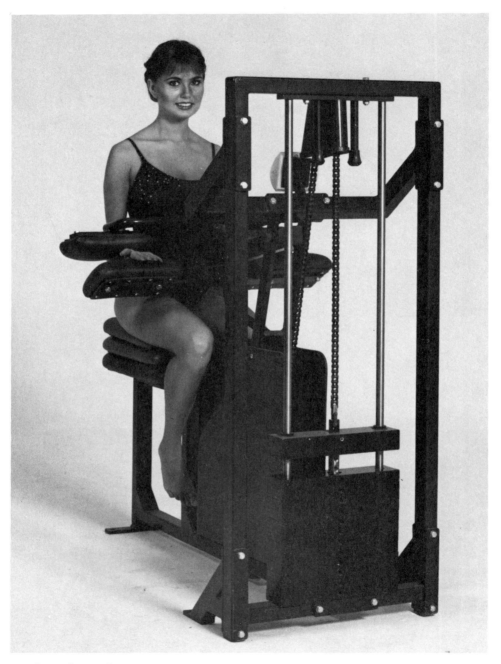

Muscle used: trapezius
Points to emphasize:
1. Place forearms between pads while seated.
2. Keep palms open and back of hands pressed against bottom pads.
3. Straighten torso until weight stack is lifted. Seat may be raised with elevation pads.

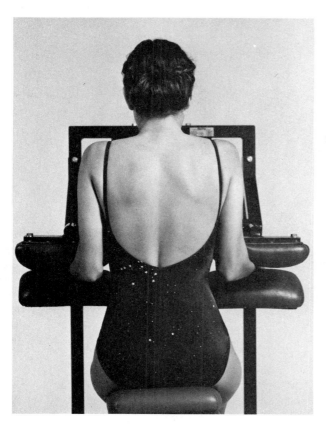

4. Elevate shoulders smoothly as high as possible. Keep elbows by sides when shrugging. Do not lean back.
5. Pause.

6. Return slowly to stretched position and repeat.

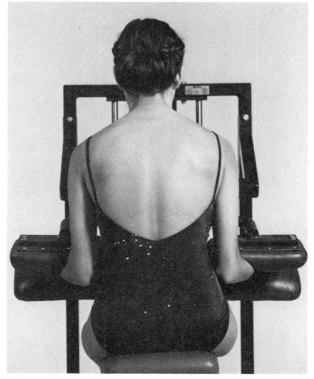

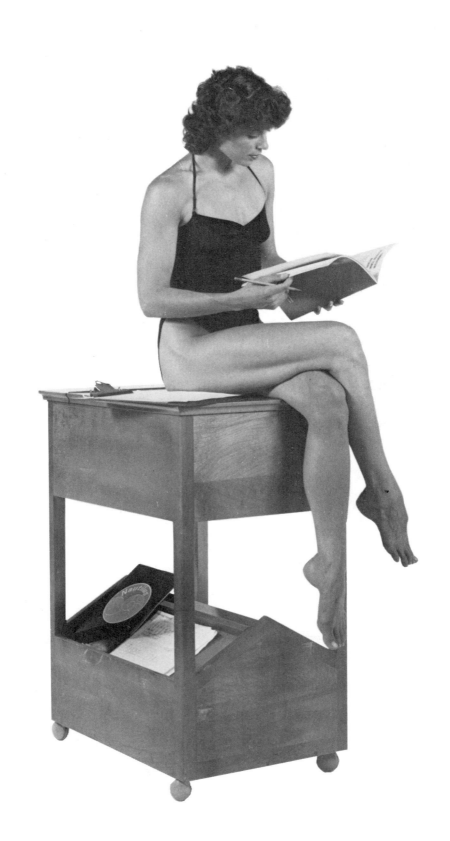

13
ROUTINES:
Basic and Specialized

The following list of exercises, grouped by body part and equipment, is a summation of the last nine chapters.

Master List of Exercises

BODY PART	NAUTILUS MACHINE OR EXERCISE
Hips	Duo Hip and Back
	Hip Abduction
	Hip Flexion
Thighs	Leg Extension
	Leg Press
	Leg Curl
	Side Leg Curl
	Duo Squat
	Hip Adduction
Calves	Calf Raise on Multi-Exercise
	Seated Calf Raise on Multi-Exercise
	Foot Flexion on Leg Curl
Back	Women's Pullover
	Pullover/Torso Arm
	Pullover
	Torso Arm Pulldown
	Behind Neck/Torso Arm
	Behind Neck
	Behind Neck Pulldown
	Behind Neck
	Lower Back

Shoulders	Double Shoulder Lateral Raise Overhead Press Lateral Raise Overhead Press 70° Shoulder Rowing Torso

Chest	Women's Chest
	Double Chest
	  Arm Cross
	  Decline Press
	Duo Decline Press
	10° Chest
	40° Chest/Shoulder

Arms	Multi-Biceps Multi-Triceps Chin on Multi-Exercise Dip on Multi-Exercise Wrist Curl on Multi-Exercise Reverse Wrist Curl on Multi-Exercise
Waist	Abdominal (Old) Abdominal (New) Rotary Torso Side Bend on Multi-Exercise
Neck	4-Way Neck Neck and Shoulder

Application of the Nautilus guidelines from Chapter 3 to the Master List of Exercises makes it possible to organize many effective routines. The following programs, divided into *basic* and *specialized,* have been used successfully by women of all ages.

Basic Nautilus Routines

The basic programs are designed to lay a foundation of strength for all major muscle groups. If certain Nautilus machines are not available, substitutions can be made.

BASIC ROUTINE 1
  1. Duo Hip and Back
  2. Hip Adduction
  3. Leg Extension
  4. Leg Curl

5. Pullover or Women's Pullover
6. Pulldown
7. Lateral Raise
8. Overhead Press
9. Neck and Shoulder
10. Arm Cross or Women's Chest
11. Decline Press
12. 4-Way Neck, Back Extension

BASIC ROUTINE 2
1. Lower Back
2. Hip Abduction
3. Leg Extension
4. Calf Raise
5. Behind Neck
6. Behind Neck Pulldown
7. Negative Dip
8. Rowing Torso
9. Multi-Triceps Extension
10. Multi-Biceps Curl
11. Abdominal
12. Neck and Shoulder

BASIC ROUTINE 3
1. Leg Curl or Side Leg Curl
2. Hip Adduction
3. Leg Press or Duo Squat
4. Hip Flexion
5. Pullover or Women's Pullover
6. Overhead Press
7. Negative Chin
8. Negative Dip
9. Wrist Curl
10. Reverse Wrist Curl
11. Abdominal
12. Rotary Torso

BASIC ROUTINE 4
1. Hip Flexion
2. Leg Extension
3. Leg Press or Duo Squat

    4. Leg Curl
    5. Calf Raise
    6. Lateral Raise
    7. Overhead Press
    8. Pullover or Women's Pullover
    9. Pulldown
   10. Arm Cross or Women's Chest
   11. Decline Press or Duo Decline Press
   12. Neck and Shoulder

BASIC ROUTINE 5
    1. Hip Adduction
    2. Hip Abduction
    3. Duo Hip and Back
    4. Hip Flexion
    5. Behind Neck
    6. Negative Chin
    7. Decline Press
    8. Rowing Torso
    9. Multi-Triceps Extension
   10. Multi-Biceps Curl
   11. Abdominal
   12. Lower Back

BASIC ROUTINE 6
    1. Leg Press or Duo Squat
    2. Leg Extension
    3. Calf Raise
    4. Lower Back
    5. Leg Curl or Side Leg Curl
    6. Lateral Raise
    7. Pullover
    8. Decline Press or Duo Decline Press
    9. Wrist Curl
   10. Reverse Wrist Curl
   11. 4-Way Neck, Lateral Contraction Right and Left
   12. Rotary Torso

Most women will get excellent results by performing Basic Routine 1 three times a week for the first month. After the first month of Routine 1, you may start alternating 1 with 2, 3, 4, 5, and 6. After three more months of training you should be able to devise your own routines by applying the guidelines from Chapter 3.

Specialized Nautilus Routines

Many women have an area of the body—such as the hips, thighs, chest, or waist—that merits special attention. If you have a problem area, then the routines below may offer a solution. Two workouts are listed for each body part. Either may be used.

Generally, most of the specialized routines are composed of seven exercises for the problem area and five exercises for the rest of your body. One of the best exercises for the problem body part is usually done for two sets. Frequently, the best exercise is performed first and last in the routine.

Two sets of a Nautilus exercise in the same workout are seldom a proficient way to shape and strengthen the body. But by performing the same exercise first and last in the routine, a slightly different degree of muscle-fiber recruitment is involved. This seems to stimulate additional firming and toning in the problem area.

An important concept to understand in using the specialized Nautilus programs is that the body will tolerate only a limited amount of disproportionate training. Women who want to strengthen and shape the thighs, for example, will accomplish this more efficiently by training all the major parts of the body, not just the thighs. From this standpoint, a specialized routine should not be used more than two times a week.

A specialized routine might be performed on Monday and Friday of a given week. But one of the basic routines should be practiced on Wednesday.

A woman with several problem areas, such as the hips and waist, might perform a specialized routine for the hips on Monday, a specialized routine for the waist on Wednesday, and a basic routine for the entire body on Friday. Regardless of the number of problem areas that a woman may have, she should always adhere to at least one basic workout per week. This will assure the best possible bodyshaping results.

Important note: Women who train on Nautilus equipment in commercial fitness centers should make certain that they have the management's approval before any listed routine is tried. Under some circumstances, it is neither practical nor advisable to perform certain exercises or routines.

SPECIALIZED ROUTINE 1: HIPS AND BUTTOCKS
1. Hip Abduction
2. Duo Hip and Back
3. Hip Flexion
4. Duo Squat or Leg Press
5. Leg Curl
6. Leg Extension
7. Lower Back
8. Pullover or Women's Pullover
9. Lateral Raise
10. Behind Neck Pulldown
11. Decline Press
12. Hip Abduction

SPECIALIZED ROUTINE 2: HIPS AND BUTTOCKS
1. Leg Curl or Side Leg Curl
2. Duo Hip and Back
3. Duo Squat or Leg Press
4. Hip Abduction
5. Hip Adduction
6. Hip Abduction
7. Arm Cross or Women's Chest
8. Overhead Press
9. Neck and Shoulder
10. Abdominal
11. Rotary Torso
12. Duo Squat or Leg Press

SPECIALIZED ROUTINE 3: THIGHS
1. Leg Extension
2. Leg Press or Duo Squat
3. Leg Curl
4. Hip Abduction
5. Hip Adduction
6. Hip Flexion
7. Pullover
8. Torso Arm Pulldown
9. Arm Cross
10. Decline Press
11. Leg Extension
12. Leg Curl

SPECIALIZED ROUTINE 4: THIGHS
1. Hip Adduction
2. Leg Extension
3. Hip Abduction
4. Leg Curl or Side Leg Curl
5. Duo Squat or Leg Press
6. Duo Hip and Back
7. Leg Extension
8. Decline Press
9. Rowing Torso
10. Multi-Biceps Curl
11. Multi-Triceps Extension
12. Hip Adduction

SPECIALIZED ROUTINE 5: CALVES
1. Calf Raise
2. Foot Flexion
3. Seated Calf Raise
4. Leg Curl
5. Duo Squat or Leg Press
6. Lateral Raise
7. Overhead Press
8. Behind Neck
9. Behind Neck Pulldown
10. Rowing Torso
11. Calf Raise
12. Foot Flexion

SPECIALIZED ROUTINE 6: CALVES
1. Duo Hip and Back
2. Leg Extension
3. Leg Curl
4. Calf Raise
5. Foot Flexion
6. Calf Raise
7. Foot Flexion
8. Arm Cross
9. Decline Press
10. Pullover
11. Rowing Torso
12. Torso Arm Pulldown

SPECIALIZED ROUTINE 7: BACK
1. Pullover or Women's Pullover
2. Behind Neck
3. Behind Neck Pulldown
4. Rowing Torso
5. Arm Cross or Women's Chest
6. Lateral Raise
7. Lower Back
8. Abdominal
9. Duo Hip and Back
10. Rotary Torso
11. Leg Extension
12. Pullover or Women's Pullover

SPECIALIZED ROUTINE 8: BACK
1. Behind Neck
2. Behind Neck Pulldown
3. Pullover or Women's Pullover
4. Torso Arm Pulldown
5. Decline Press
6. Neck and Shoulder
7. 4-Way Neck, Back Extension
8. Lower Back
9. Hip Abduction
10. Hip Adduction
11. Negative Dip
12. Negative Chin

SPECIALIZED ROUTINE 9: SHOULDERS
1. Lateral Raise
2. Overhead Press
3. Rowing Torso
4. Decline Press
5. Neck and Shoulder
6. 70° Shoulder
7. Pullover or Women's Pullover
8. Leg Extension
9. Leg Curl
10. Multi-Biceps Curl
11. Multi-Triceps Extension
12. Lateral Raise

SPECIALIZED ROUTINE 10: SHOULDERS
1. Overhead Press
2. 70° Shoulder
3. Behind Neck Pulldown
4. Lateral Raise
5. Decline Press
6. 40° Chest/Shoulder
7. Negative Chin
8. Negative Dip
9. Hip Adduction
10. Hip Abduction
11. Duo Squat or Leg Press
12. Overhead Press

SPECIALIZED ROUTINE 11: CHEST
1. Arm Cross or Women's Chest
2. Decline Press or Duo Decline Press
3. Pullover or Women's Pullover
4. 40° Chest/Shoulder
5. Rowing Torso
6. Lateral Raise
7. Behind Neck Pulldown
8. Leg Extension
9. Leg Curl
10. Calf Raise
11. Abdominal
12. Decline Press or Duo Decline Press

SPECIALIZED ROUTINE 12: CHEST
1. 40° Chest/Shoulder
2. Negative Dip
3. 10° Chest
4. Decline Press or Duo Decline Press
5. Pullover or Women's Pullover
6. Leg Extension
7. Leg Press or Squat
8. 70° Shoulder
9. Duo Hip and Back
10. Hip Abduction
11. Multi-Biceps Curl
12. 40° Chest/Shoulder

SPECIALIZED ROUTINE 13: ARMS
1. Multi-Biceps Curl
2. Behind Neck Pulldown
3. Multi-Triceps Extension
4. Decline Press
5. Lateral Raise
6. Rowing Torso
7. Pullover or Women's Pullover
8. Overhead Press
9. Leg Extension
10. Leg Curl
11. Wrist Curl
12. Reverse Wrist Curl

SPECIALIZED ROUTINE 14: ARMS
1. Negative Dip
2. Negative Chin
3. Multi-Biceps Curl
4. Multi-Triceps Extension
5. Wrist Curl
6. Reverse Wrist Curl
7. Duo Hip and Back
8. Hip Flexion
9. Lower Back
10. Abdominal
11. Decline Press or Duo Decline Press
12. Torso Arm Pulldown

SPECIALIZED ROUTINE 15: WAIST
1. Side Bend
2. Rotary Torso
3. Abdominal
4. Hip Flexion
5. Leg Extension
6. Leg Press
7. Neck and Shoulder
8. Hip Abduction
9. Calf Raise
10. Lower Back
11. Decline Press
12. Pullover or Women's Pullover

SPECIALIZED ROUTINE 16: WAIST
1. Abdominal
2. Rotary Torso
3. Hip Flexion
4. Duo Hip and Back
5. Pullover or Women's Pullover
6. Overhead Press
7. Arm Cross or Women's Chest
8. Leg Extension
9. Leg Curl
10. Duo Squat
11. Abdominal
12. Rotary Torso

SPECIALIZED ROUTINE 17: NECK
1. Leg Curl
2. Leg Extension
3. Hip Adduction
4. Hip Abduction
5. Pullover or Women's Pullover
6. Rowing Torso
7. Lateral Raise
8. Overhead Press
9. 4-Way Neck, Front and Back
10. 4-Way Neck, Lateral Contraction Right and Left
11. Rotary Neck
12. Neck and Shoulder

Using the Nautilus
Training Record (pp. 158-61)

A GRADUAL INTRODUCTION

For best results, a beginning trainee should undergo a two-week introduction to Nautilus equipment. Rather than performing all the exercises of Basic Routine 1, she is advised to begin her first workout with only five simple machines. A good choice would be hip adduction, leg extension, leg curl, pullover, and decline press. Add one or two new machines each workout until all 12 exercises of Basic Routine 1 are being utilized. A gradual two-week introduction to Nautilus machines ensures proper form on each exercise.

AFTER THE FIRST WEEK

The duo hip and back is often a difficult machine for a beginner to use. It should be introduced after the third workout.

The overhead press on the double shoulder machine, because of its difficulty, should be initiated after the lateral raise is mastered.

The 4-way neck machine, since it provides exercise for the vulnerable cervical area of the spine, should be introduced last.

HIGHER REPETITIONS

On the duo hip and back and duo squat machines, it is permissable to use 15 to 20 repetitions for each leg rather than the standard 8 to 12 repetitions.

RECORD KEEPING

Several methods have been employed successfully by Nautilus Fitness Centers to record the resistance that the trainee uses on each Nautilus machine. The method on p. 146 labels the weight stack in 10-pound increments. (Other ways include numbering and lettering the weight plates.) The top plate, which includes the selector rod, weighs 20 pounds. Thus, the plates would be individually labeled in ascending order from 20 to 150 pounds or more.

For example, the first entry recorded on the decline press is 30/8. This indicates that the trainee performed 30 pounds for 8 repetitions. Fourteen repetitions with 30 pounds were performed during the third workout, so the resistance was increased approximately 5 percent for workout four. This was accomplished by the addition of a small 1.25-pound saddle plate to the top of the weight stack.

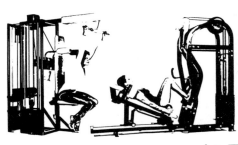
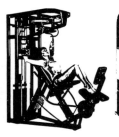
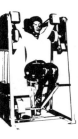
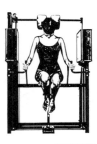

Nautilus Training Record

name _____

	date	6/3	6/5	6/7	6/10	6/12	6/14	6/17	6/19	6/21
BASIC ROUTINE 1										
Hips										
1. Duo Hip and Back		40/18	40/19	40/20	42.5/15	42.5/16	42.5/18	42.5/19	42.5/22	45/15
2. Hip Adduction		30/8	30/10	30/12	31.25/9	31.25/10	31.25/11	31.25/12	32.5/8	32.5/10
Thighs										
3. Leg Extension		35/9	35/11	35/13	37.5/8	37.5/9	37.5/9	37/5/10	37.5/11	37.5/14
4. Leg Curl		20/11	20/12	21.25/10	21.25/11	21.25/13	22.5/8	22.5/9	22.5/10	22.5/11
Back										
5. Women' Pullover		40/10	40/10	40/12	42.5/9	42.5/11	42.5/12	45/7	45/8	45/9
6. Pulldown		30/7	30/9	30/8	30/10	30/11	30/14	31.25/10	31.25/10	31.25/11
Shoulders										
7. Lateral Raise		20/13	21.25/6	21.25/7	21.25/8	21.25/9	21.25/9	21.25/11	21.25/12	22.5/8
8. Overhead Press		20/8	20/8	20/6	20/8	20/9	20/9	20/11	20/11	20/12
9. Neck and Shoulder		20/9	20/8	20/9	20/11	20/13	21.25/10	21.25/10	21.25/11	21.25/12
Chest										
10. Women's Chest		30/12	31.25/9	31.25/10	31.25/10	31.25/12	32.5/9	32.5/8	32.5/9	32.5/
11. Decline Press		30/8	30/9	30/14	31.25/8	31.25/9	31.25/11	31.25/12	32.5/8	32.5/9
Neck										
12. 4-Way Neck		20/10	20/11	20/11	20/13	21.25/8	21.25/9	21.25/10	21.25/11	21.25/12

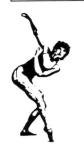
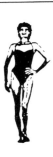
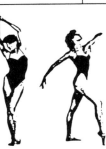
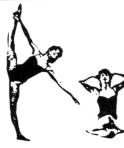
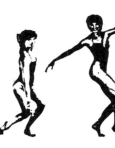

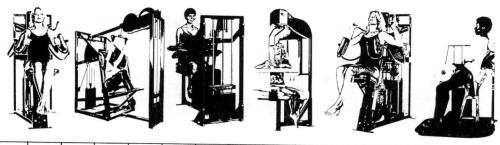

A blank Nautilus Training Record is provided for your use on the following two pages.

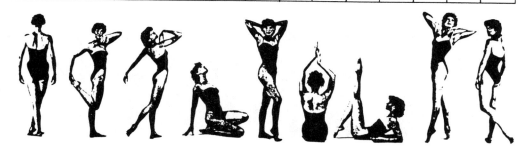

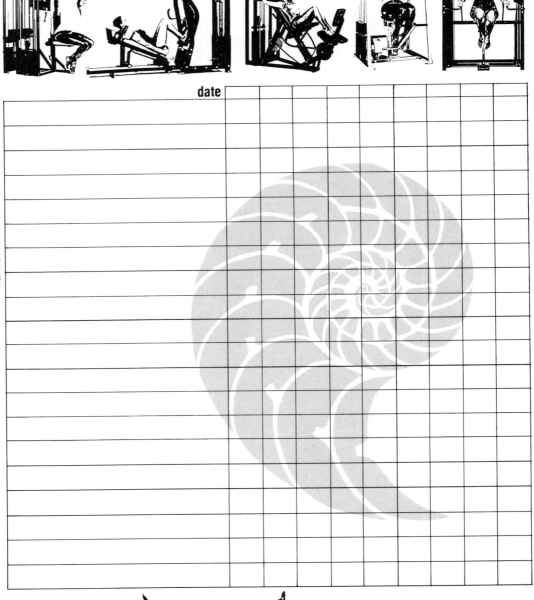

Nautilus Training Record

name

date

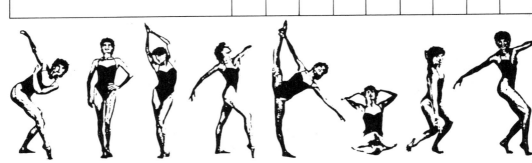

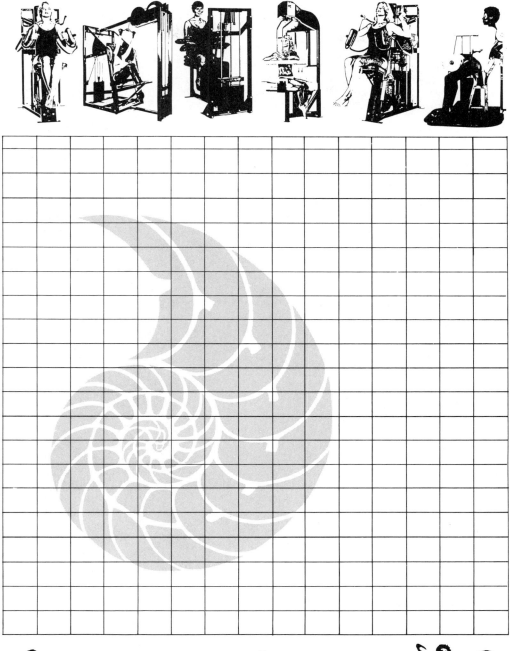
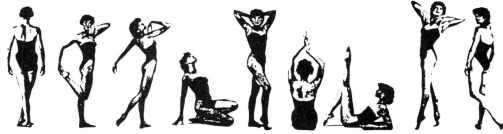

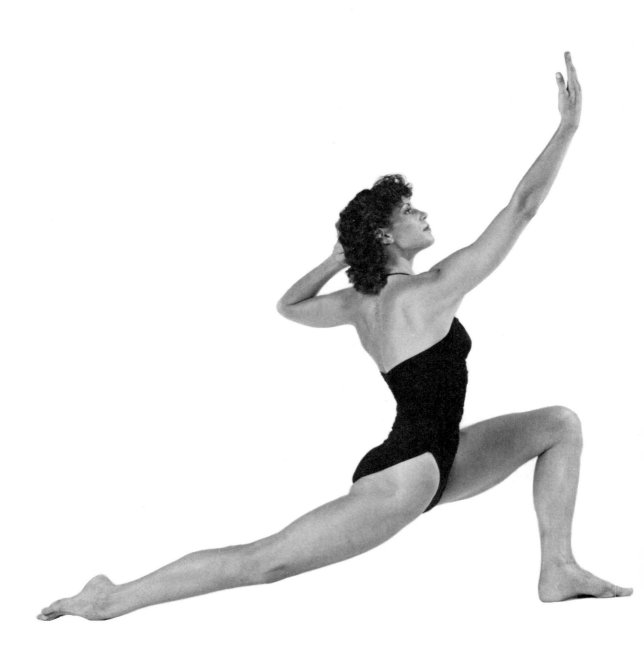

14
COMPETITION:
Bodybuilding with Nautilus

Competitive bodybuilding for women is booming. In 1979, the only two organized contests for women enlisted a mere 40 competitors! During 1985 there were at least 400 shows attracting over 12,000 entrants. The most coveted title, Ms. Olympia, is awarded each year in November with at least $10,000 in prize money going to the winner.

Bodybuilding contests are judged on three basic components: *muscularity*—shape, development, and definition of individual muscles and muscle groups: *symmetry*—overall back to front proportion and balance of upper body compared to lower; and *presentation*—a 90-second posing routine performed with music. A successful routine includes a wide variety of artistic and muscular poses, all connected with transitions featuring gymnastics and dance movements.

A bodybuilder's presentation and posing are improved through practice and coaching. Both muscularity and symmetry are developed through proper exercise. Definition or clarity of the superficial muscles is a result of removing the layer of fat that normally lies between the skin and the muscles. Reducing subcutaneous fat requires a long-duration, lower-calorie diet combined with exercise.

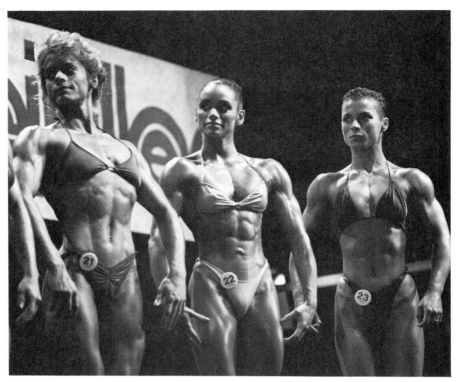

Much of a bodybuilder's symmetry is judged by making group comparisons from the front, side, and back. Above and below are several contestants from the 1984 Ms. Olympia: (above) Carla Temple, Gladys Portugues and Erica Mes; (below) Carla Dunlap and winner Cory Everson.

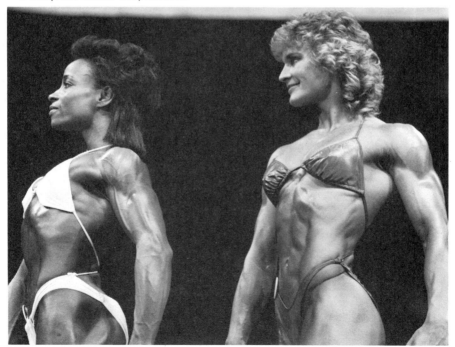

The Importance of Genetics

The basic training of a bodybuilder should be no different than the training of most fitness-minded women. The primary differences are not in the training, but in the ways the successful bodybuilder responds to the training.

Successful women bodybuilders have more genetic potential for bodybuilding than do most women. Desired physical characteristics are long muscle bellies, broad shoulders, narrow hips, and a low-level of subcutaneous fat. All of these characteristics are inherited and are not subject to positive modification. Women who possess these characteristics, however, get faster and better bodybuilding results from their training.

Motivation for Bodybuilding

While competitive bodybuilding is certainly not for all fitness-minded women, there is no doubt that it motivates some.

"I think the main motivation is seeing the fruits of your labors," says Rachel McLish, two-time winner of Ms. Olympia. "Most women start seeing improvement in their bodies within two weeks. Everybody wants muscles, whether they know it or not. When you use words like 'tone' and 'tighten' and 'firm,' you're talking muscles."

"Bodybuilding is actually a tool for prolonged youth—at least, the muscle tone and body composition that we identify with youth," Carla Dunlap, 1983 Ms. Olympia, writes in a recent issue of *Muscle and Fitness*. "Women are discovering the marvelous benefits of exercise in greater and greater numbers, but they are just beginning to appreciate the unique benefits of bodybuilding."

Both Rachel McLish and Carla Dunlap would agree that successful bodybuilding requires resistance exercise, and resistance exercise entails an understanding and application of *intensity, progression,* and *form.* These three principles also make up the backbone of Nautilus training. Nautilus training, therefore, is an efficient method of bodybuilding for dedicated women.

Nautilus exercise will help any bodybuilder reach her goals faster. In fact, two courses—*The Nautilus Bodybuilding Book* and *The Nautilus Advanced Bodybuilding Book*—have been published especially for bodybuilders. Included in these books are Nautilus routines that apply to both men and women.

Before several bodybuilding routines are described, it is important to reinforce some of the facts discussed in Chapter 2 on muscles.

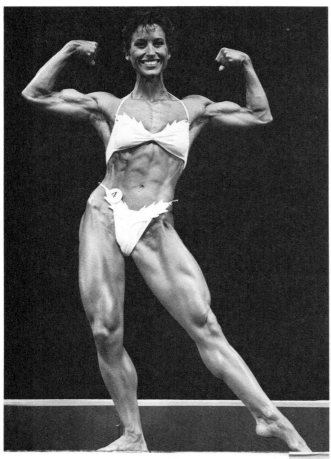

Rachel McLish is five-feet-six-inches tall and weighs 120 pounds. "Muscle," Rachel says, "is the key to building an attractive body."

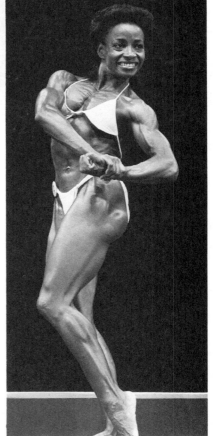

Carla Dunlap knows the importance of a lean, strong body.

More About Muscles

Many women, no doubt, are still concerned that they will become overly developed through bodybuilding training. The truth is that building larger muscles is very difficult for most people regardless of gender. Women are born with fewer muscle fibers than men and a different hormone balance. Thus, it is impossible for most women to build muscle mass rapidly.

Be aware, too, that the process is reversible. Should you ever think you are too muscular, merely cut back on your training and the extra mass will disappear. You will find that atrophy is all too easy to achieve.

There are, however, a few women who have unusual talent and the necessary genetic make-up for building muscle, women who go beyond bodybuilding for fitness and take it up as a profession. They dedicate themselves to the total pursuit of the ultimate physique. Such total pursuit also includes the adherence to a strict diet for many months to become very lean.

Many champion bodybuilders, such as Rachel McLish, Carla Dunlap, Julie McNew, Gladys Portugues, Lynne Pirie, Lori Bowen-Rice, and Cory Everson, use Nautilus frequently in their training. They've found that Nautilus allows them to isolate certain muscles and work those muscles more efficiently than is possible using barbells and dumbbells.

An especially productive form of bodybuilding exercise performed with Nautilus equipment is called pre-exhaustion. A close examination of it is in order.

Pre-Exhaustion

Barbell exercises, such as the squat, bench press, and overhead press, share a common problem: In any exercise where two or more muscle groups are involved, a point of exhaustion is reached when the weakest group is no longer able to continue. In this case, very little muscle stimulation is provided for the stronger muscles involved in the same exercise.

In the barbell bench press, for example, a point of failure is usually reached when the triceps muscles become fatigued. This normally happens before the larger and stronger pectoral muscles have been worked as hard as necessary to produce the best-possible results. But by pre-exhausting the pectorals the problem can be solved.

To pre-exhaust the pectorals, a bodybuilder would first perform a set of straight-armed flies with dumbbells, and immediately follow

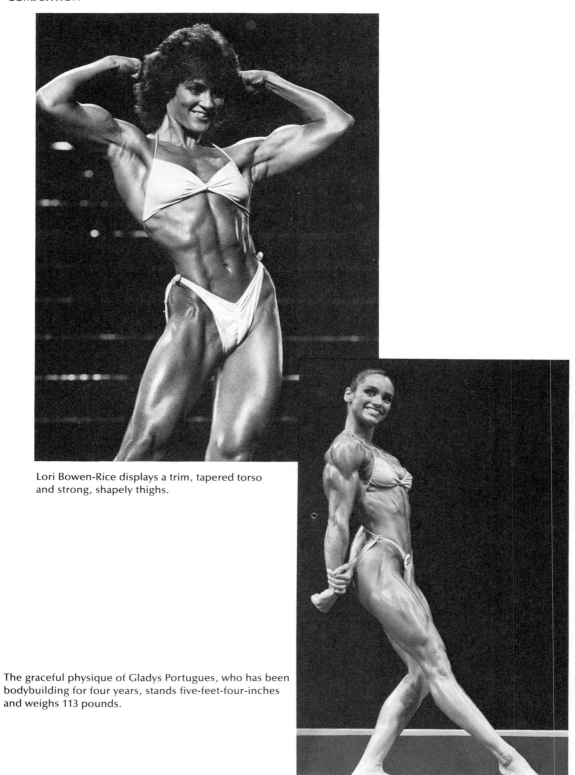

Lori Bowen-Rice displays a trim, tapered torso and strong, shapely thighs.

The graceful physique of Gladys Portugues, who has been bodybuilding for four years, stands five-feet-four-inches and weighs 113 pounds.

this with a set of barbell bench presses. By moving instantly from the flies to the presses, the triceps of the arms are temporarily stronger than the pectorals of the chest. Thus, the triceps can now force the normally stronger pectorals to a new level of growth stimulation.

While such pre-exhaustion training can be used to make conventional exercise more efficient, it is even more productive when used with certain Nautilus machines. At least five Nautilus double machines are specifically designed to be performed in a pre-exhaustion manner:

Compound Leg—leg extensions followed by leg presses.

Pullover/Torso Arm—pullovers followed by pulldowns to chest.

Behind Neck/Torso Arm—behind necks followed by behind neck pulldowns.

Double Shoulder—lateral raises followed by overhead presses.

Double Chest—arm crosses followed by decline presses.

All the preceding Nautilus machines involve a single-joint rotary primary movement plus a multiple-joint compound secondary movement. It is very important on all pre-exhaustion exercises to move very quickly, in less than three seconds, from the end of the primary set to the beginning of the secondary set. Recovery time of the pre-exhausted muscle is a matter of only a few seconds; therefore, the time between the two exercises determines whether you get fair or maximum results.

Below are two different pre-exhaustion routines. The exercises inside the brackets are performed back-to-back with no rest in between.

Pre-Exhaustion Bodybuilding Routine A	Pre-Exhaustion Bodybuilding Routine B
1. Leg Extension	1. Hip and Back
2. Leg Press	2. Duo Squat
3. Leg Curl	3. Hip Abduction
4. Calf Raise	4. Hip Adduction
5. Pullover	5. Behind Neck
6. Pulldown	6. Behind Neck Pulldown
7. Multi-Triceps Extension	7. 10° Chest
8. Lateral Raise	8. Neck and Shoulder
9. Overhead Press	9. Multi-Biceps Curl
10. Multi-Biceps Curl	10. Negative Chin
11. Arm Cross	11. Multi-Triceps Extension
12. Decline Press	12. Negative Dip

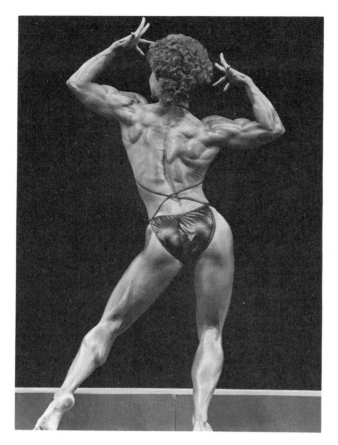

World champion Clare Furr has one of the best backs in women's bodybuilding. Her legs also are outstanding.

The pre-exhaustion routines are higher in intensity than the basic routines in Chapter 13. You should make sure that you have developed an above-average level of strength before trying them. Furthermore, you should only perform one routine or the other one time per week. The remaining two workouts should be basic.

Women bodybuilders who are at the advanced level, or who have trained seriously for at least one year, may also want to try double pre-exhaustion training..

Double Pre-Exhaustion

Normal pre-exhaustion training is performed when a single-joint movement is immediately followed by a multiple-joint movement. For example, in the compound leg machine, the leg extension

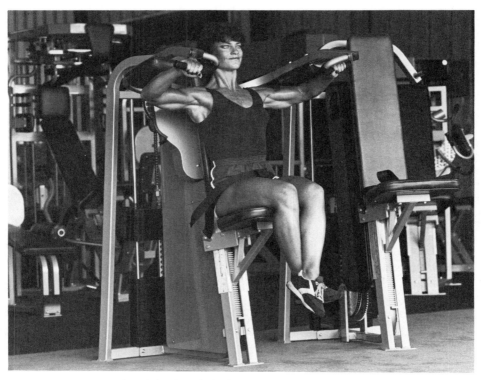

Julie McNew taxes her deltoids with the lateral raise machine.

After the lateral raise, Julie employs the overhead press to force her pre-exhausted deltoids to a deeper level of growth stimulation.

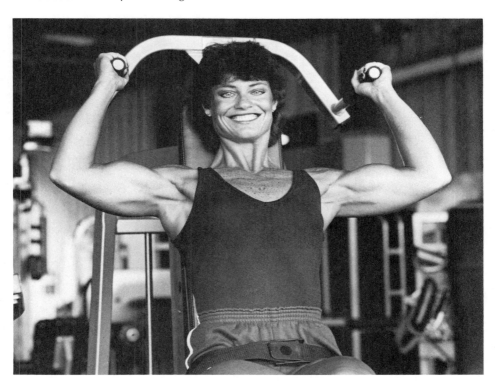

is the single-joint movement and the leg press is the multiple-joint movement. The leg extension pre-exhausts the quadriceps of the frontal thighs. Then before the frontal thighs can recover, the leg press brings into action the gluteals, hamstrings, and gastroc-soleus to force the quadriceps to a deeper state of exhaustion.

Double pre-exhaustion for the thighs goes a step further. Instead of performing two exercises back to back, you do three in a row: (1) leg press, (2) leg extension, and (3) duo squat. The most demanding exercise is always performed last in the series. Double pre-exhaustion may be applied to most major muscle groups.

Two recommended double pre-exhaustion routines are listed below. The first emphasizes the legs and the second concentrates on the arms. Once again, the exercise inside the brackets should be done with no rest in between.

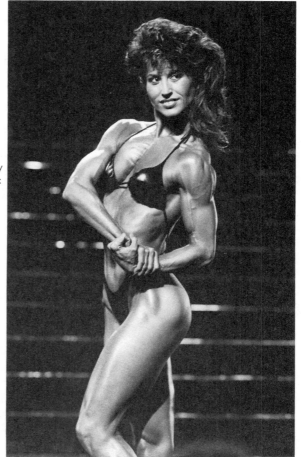

Rachel McLish demonstrates perfectly what women's bodybuilding is about: muscularity, symmetry, and presentation.

Double Pre-Exhaustion Bodybuilding Routine C—Legs

1. Leg Press
2. Leg Extension
3. Duo Squat
4. Calf Raise
5. Leg Curl
6. Hip Abduction
7. Hip and Back
8. Pullover
9. Lateral Raise
10. Behind Neck Pulldown
11. Decline Press
12. Abdominal

Double Pre-Exhaustion Bodybuilding Routine D—Arms

1. Behind Neck Pulldown
2. Multi-Biceps Curl
3. Negative Chin
4. Lower Back
5. Decline Press
6. Multi-Triceps Extension
7. Negative Dip
8. Wrist Curl
9. 10° Chest
10. Pullover
11. Neck and Shoulder
12. Duo Squat or Leg Press

Because of the unusual demands placed on your body's recovery ability, do not perform a double pre-exhaustion routine more than once a week. Remember, more is not better when it applies to high-intensity exercise.

Strive to make your exercises harder, not easier—briefer, not longer—and your bodybuilding results will be outstanding.

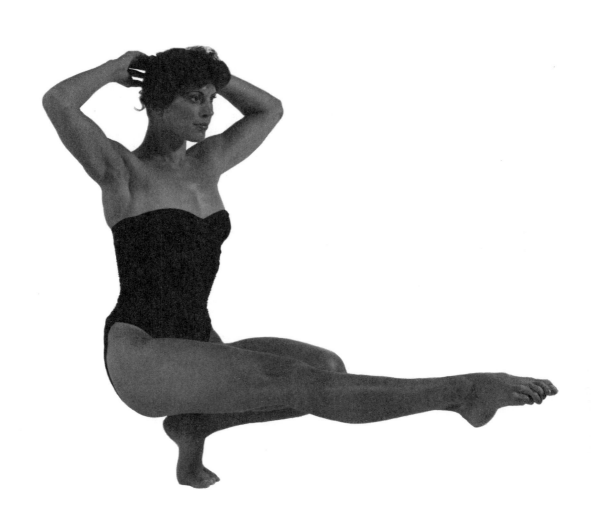

15
CALISTHENICS:
Maximizing
Freehand Exercises

What if it is not convenient for you to use Nautilus equipment on a regular basis? Can you apply the Nautilus bodyshaping rules to freehand calisthenic exercises?

Yes, indeed you can and with fairly good results.

Most calisthenic exercises can be made more productive by the use of ordinary items found around almost any household. The following items will be needed:

- 2 kitchen chairs with flat backs
- 1 strong broom handle or pipe
- 1 small bench
- 2 medium-sized cans of vegetables. They should weigh about 2 pounds each.
- 1 large can of fruit or vegetable juice
- 2 plastic bottles with sculptured handles. The 1-gallon size full of water weighs about 9 pounds. The weight can be decreased by using less water.

The two chairs can be used as parallel bars to support your body's weight in various exercises. The broomstick or pipe laid across the backs of the chairs can be a horizontal bar to support the weight of your body or to simulate a barbell. Lying across a bench often provides a more effective means of exercise than lying on the floor. The plastic bottles and cans of vegetables make excellent weights to hold in the hands.

The major problem with calisthenic-type exercises is their inability to isolate and overload a specific muscle group. Unlike Nautilus machines, calisthenics do not provide rotary, direct, balanced resistance.

Some calisthenics are much better than others, or at least they can be adapted to be more productive. The potential benefits of calisthenics or freehand exercises are largely determined by two factors: the quantity of movement by a specific part of the body and the quality of the resistance applied against it.

All of the following exercises were taken from *The Darden Technique for Weight Loss, Body Shaping and Slenderizing*. Perform them exactly as described.

SQUAT WITH PLASTIC BOTTLES

Muscles used: gluteus maximus, quadriceps, hamstrings, and gastroc-soleus group

Points to emphasize:
1. Stand erect, feet shoulder-width apart, with a bottle in each hand.
2. Lower the upper body by slowly bending the knees and hips. Look straight ahead or slightly upward during the movement. **3.** Continue downward until the back thighs come in contact with the calves. **4.** Do not relax or bounce at the bottom of the movement. **5.** Return smoothly to the starting position and repeat.

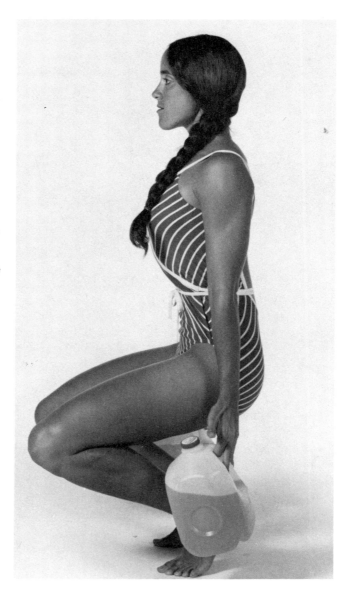

ONE-LEGGED SQUAT

Muscles used: gluteus maximus, quadriceps, hamstrings, and gastroc-soleus group
Points to emphasize:
1. Grasp the back of a straight chair with the left hand and hold the left leg in front of the body. Do not let the left foot touch the floor during the movement. **2.** Lower the upper body slowly by bending the right knee and hip. Look straight ahead or slightly upward during the movement. **3.** Continue downward until the back thigh comes in contact with the calf. **4.** Do not relax or bounce at the bottom of the movement. **5.** Return smoothly to the starting position and repeat. **6.** Work the left leg in the same manner.

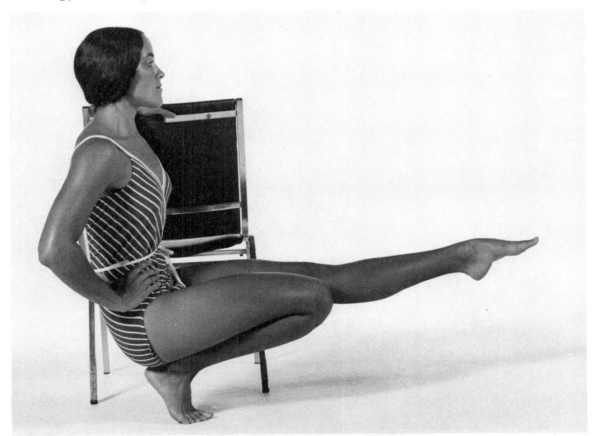

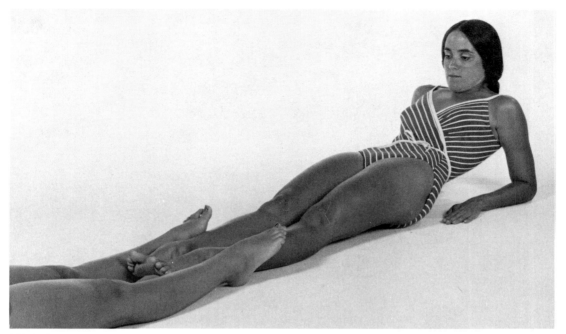

HIP ABDUCTION WITH PARTNER

Muscle used: gluteus medius
Points to emphasize:
1. Sit on floor facing a partner. Both should lean back on hands or elbows for support. **2.** Place ankles inside of partner's ankles. Keep the legs straight. **3.** Push legs laterally against partner's squeezing resistance. Partner should allow positive and negative work of this spreading function. This is felt in the outer hip. **4.** Repeat until fatigued.

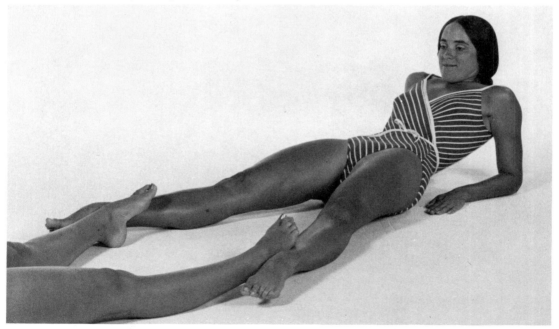

HIP ADDUCTION WITH PARTNER

Muscles used: adductor group
Points to emphasize:
1. Sit on floor facing a partner. Both should lean back on hands or elbows for support. **2.** Place ankles outside of partner's ankles. Keep legs straight. **3.** Squeeze legs forcibly together against partner's attempt to spread them. The partner provides both positive and negative resistance, which is felt in the groin and inner thigh area. **4.** Repeat until fatigued.

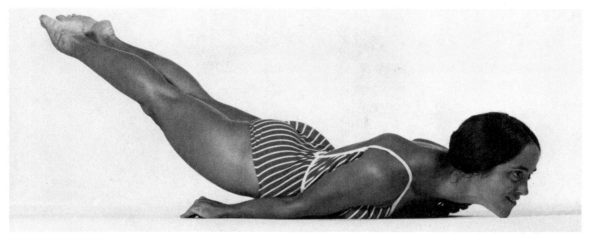

REVERSE LEG RAISE

Muscle used: gluteus maximus
Points to emphasize:
1. Lie face down on floor. **2.** Place hands by hips. **3.** Lift both legs backward as high as possible. **4.** Pause briefly at highest position and squeeze buttocks together. **5.** Return legs slowly to floor and repeat.

ONE-LEGGED CALF RAISE WITH PLASTIC BOTTLE

Muscle used: gastrocnemius
Points to emphasize:
1. Place ball of right foot on edge of a block or stair step. **2.** Lock knee and suspend other foot. **3.** Grasp a water-filled bottle in one hand and balance body with other by grasping a chair or stair rail. **4.** Raise heel as high as possible. **5.** Pause. **6.** Lower slowly to a deep stretch. **7.** Repeat until fatigued. **8.** Follow same procedure for left calf.

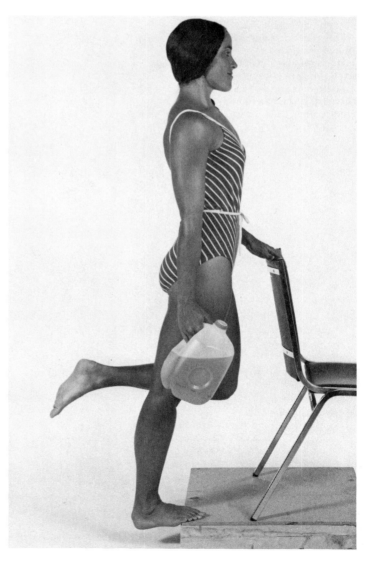

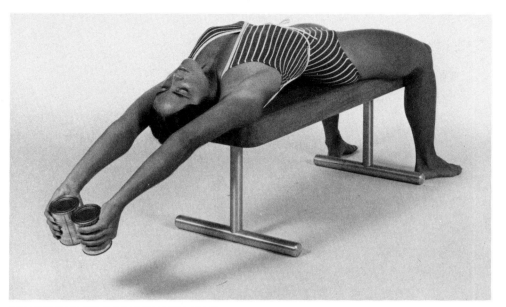

STRAIGHT-ARMED PULLOVER WITH CANS

Muscle used: latissimus dorsi
Points to emphasize:
1. Lie face up on a bench. Head
should be extended over end and feet
should be on floor. **2.** Hold cans over
chest in straight-armed position.
3. Lower weight slowly behind head.
4. Stretch. **5.** Return smoothly to over-
chest position. **6.** Repeat.

SHOULDER SHRUG WITH PLASTIC BOTTLES

Muscles used: trapezius
Points to emphasize:
1. Grasp bottles and stand. **2.** Shrug
shoulders as high as possible while
keeping arms straight. **3.** Pause in top
position. **4.** Lower slowly and repeat.

BENT-OVER ROW WITH PLASTIC BOTTLES

Muscles used: biceps and latissimus dorsi
Points to emphasize:
1. Bend at waist and grasp two plastic bottles. **2.** Keep torso parallel to floor. **3.** Pull hands upward until they touch lower chest area. **4.** Pause. **5.** Return slowly to starting position and repeat.

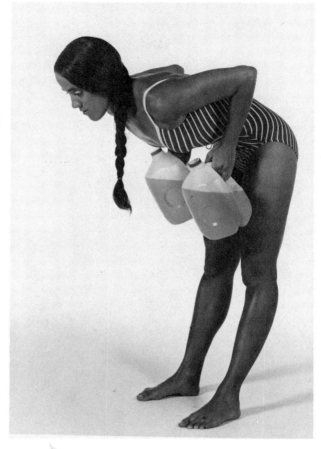

LATERAL RAISE WITH CANS

Muscle used: deltoid
Points to emphasize:
1. Stand erect with a can in each hand. **2.** Keep arms straight. **3.** Raise cans laterally to shoulder height. **4.** Pause. **5.** Lower slowly and repeat.

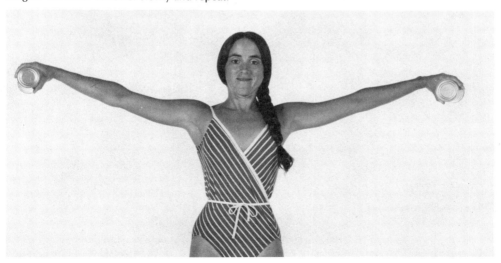

NEGATIVE CHAIR DIP

Muscles used: triceps, deltoid, and
pectoralis major
Points to emphasize:
1. Face two chairs away from each
other. **2.** Stand between them.
3. Support your body on straightened
arms against the backs of chairs.
4. Lower body slowly by bending
arms. **5.** Stretch in bottom position.
6. Place feet on floor and quickly stand
to straight-armed position. **7.** Repeat
the slow lowering movements until
fatigued.

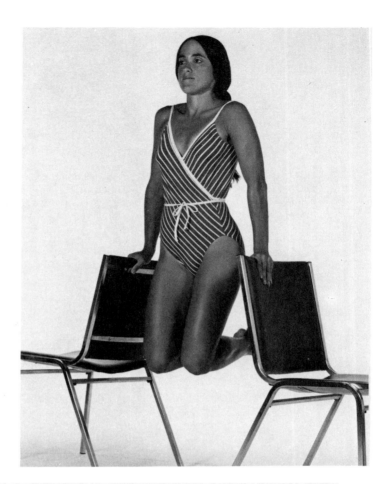

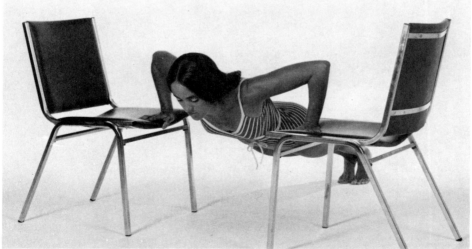

PUSHUP BETWEEN CHAIRS

Muscles used: triceps, deltoid, and pectoralis major
Points to emphasize:
1. Position two chairs so they face each other and their edges are shoulder-width apart.
2. Place each hand on one of chair seats. Arms should be straight. **3.** Hold body rigid as it
is supported on hands and toes. **4.** Lower slowly by bending arms. **5.** Push back to top
position by straightening arms. **6.** Repeat.

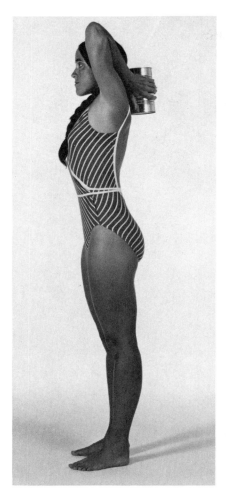

TRICEPS EXTENSION WITH CAN

Muscle used: triceps
Points to emphasize:
1. Hold a large can in the middle with both hands and raise it overhead. **2.** Keep elbows by ears. **3.** Lower the can slowly behind neck to middle of back. Do not move elbows. **4.** Raise can smoothly back to top position. **5.** Repeat.

SEATED ONE-ARMED CURL WITH CAN

Muscle used: biceps
Points to emphasize:
1. Sit on edge of a chair. **2.** Grasp large can in the right hand. **3.** Lean forward and stabilize right elbow by planting it on inside surface of right thigh. Let the arm hang. **4.** Curl can to shoulder. **5.** Lower slowly and repeat. **6.** Work left arm in same manner.

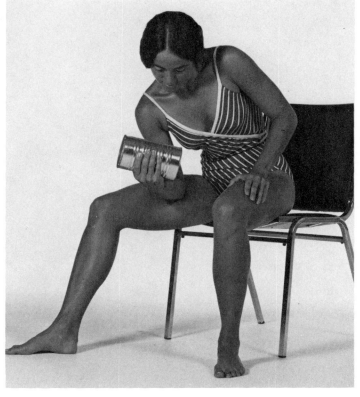

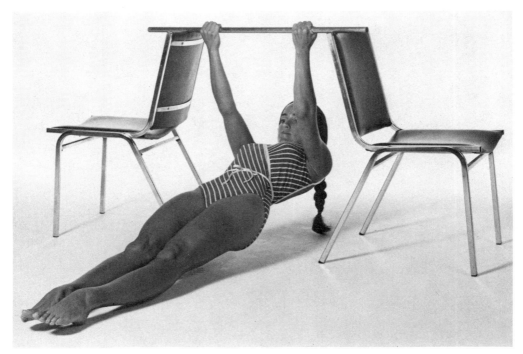

LYING CHINUP

Muscles used: biceps and latissimus
dorsi
Points to emphasize:
1. Span an approximate two-foot
distance between two chairs with a
broom handle or pipe across the
backs. 2. Position upper body under
pipe. 3. Grasp pipe with palms up.
4. Pull chest to pipe. 5. Pause and
lower slowly. Only heels should touch
floor. 6. Repeat.

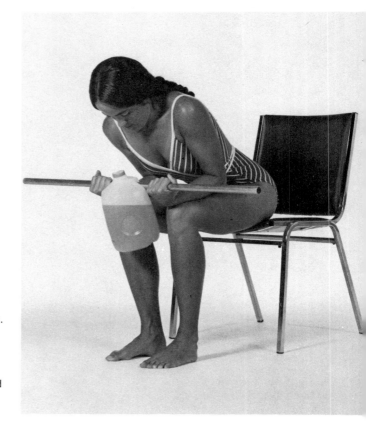

WRIST CURL WITH PLASTIC BOTTLE

Muscles used: wrist flexors
Points to emphasize:
1. Slide bottle to middle of broom handle or pipe.
2. Grasp pipe with palms up on both sides of
bottle. 3. Rest forearms on thighs and back of
hands against the knees and be seated. 4. Lean
forward until angle between upper arms and
forearms is less than 90 degrees. 5. Curl pipe and
contract forearm muscles. 6. Pause and lower
resistance slowly. 7. Repeat.

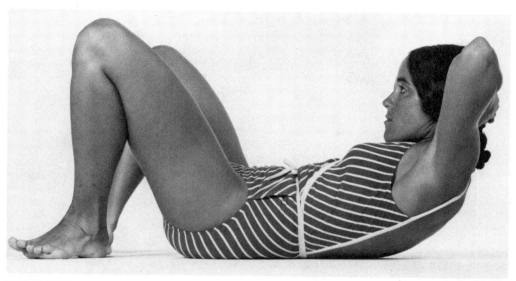

TRUNK CURL

Muscle used: rectus abdominis
Points to emphasize:
1. Lie face up on floor with hands behind head. **2.** Bring heels close to buttocks and widen knees. **3.** Try to curl trunk to a sitting position. Only one-third of a standard situp can be performed in this fashion. **4.** Pause in contracted position. **5.** Lower slowly to floor and repeat.

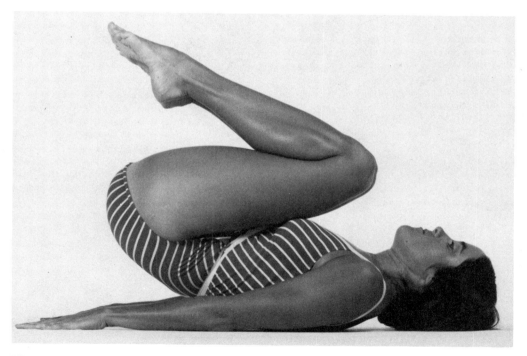

REVERSE TRUNK CURL

Muscle used: rectus abdominis
Points to emphasize:
1. Lie face-up on floor with hands on either side of hips. **2.** Bring thighs on chest so knees and hips are in a flexed position. **3.** Curl pelvic area toward chin by lifting buttocks and lower back. **4.** Pause. **5.** Lower buttocks slowly and repeat.

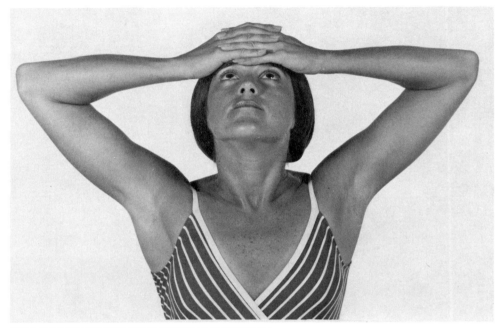

FRONT NECK FLEXION AGAINST HAND RESISTANCE

Muscle used: sternocleidomastoid
Points to emphasize:
1. Interlace fingers and place hands on forehead. **2.** Move head forward against resistance of hands and arms. When chin is on chest, use arms to push head backward. **3.** Continue this forward and backward motion until neck is fatigued.

Examples of tried-and-proved calisthenic routines are as follows:

PROGRAM 1
1. Squat with bottles
2. Hip adduction with partner
3. Hip abduction with partner
4. Straight-armed pullover with cans
5. Lying chinup
6. Negative chair dip
7. Seated one-armed curl with can
8. Triceps extension with can
9. Wrist curl
10. Trunk curl
11. Reverse trunk curl
12. Front neck flexion

PROGRAM 2
1. One-legged squat
2. Reverse leg raise
3. Hip abduction with partner
4. Hip adduction with partner
5. One-legged calf raise
6. Shoulder shrug with bottles
7. Pushup between chairs
8. Bent-over row with bottles
9. Lateral raise with cans
10. Triceps extension with can
11. Lying chinup
12. Trunk curl

Calisthenic Programs 1 and 2 can be used in the privacy of your home or even adapted for use in a hotel room as you travel. Always adhere to the rules that are stated in Chapter 3 in designing your routine.

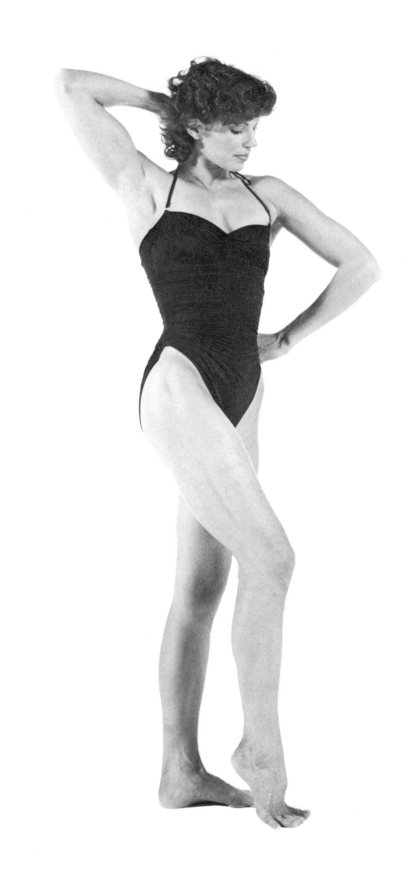

16
QUESTIONS:
Facts into Practice

The best way to fill in gaps and clear up areas of confusion from previous chapters is the simple method of questions and answers. Let us put scientific facts into practice.

Benefits of Nautilus Exercise

Q. *After reading Chapter 1, I get the impression that women should train to become more physically attractive. Is that correct?*

A. Proper exercise will make a woman more physically attractive, and many women train for that specific reason. But increased physical attractiveness is only one of the benefits of Nautilus exercise. A woman who trains properly can expect to:

- Improve her muscular strength
- Increase her joint flexibility
- Improve the function of her heart and lungs
- Develop better posture
- Develop a positive self-image
- Become more proficient in almost any sport
- Augment her energy
- Recuperate faster than average from illness or injury
- Look and feel better by shaping her muscles to their maximum potential

Whatever your goals are in the physical realm, proper exercise on Nautilus equipment will help you achieve them in the most efficient manner.

Physical Attractiveness

Q. *I'm upset that it is the outside appearance of a woman's body that primarily attracts a man. Can't something be done to correct this situation?*

A. Rest assured that there are other people who are concerned as well. Being upset, however, does not change the social behavior of most Americans.

The April, 1982, issue of *Glamour* Magazine reported the results of a survey that asked women the following question: "Have you ever felt people responded to you solely on the basis of your looks?"

"Yes," said a resounding 92 percent of the women who answered the survey.

"I've been rejected and even ostracized because of my physical appearance," wrote one concerned woman. "It seems that being overweight cancels five years of college and fluency in four languages."

"I'm fairly attractive," wrote another woman, "and at times become disgusted with men who tell me, 'You're very attractive, and I'd like to get to know you better.' What ever happened to intelligence and charm?"

Intelligence and charm are still desirable attributes, but according to the research of Dr. Ellen Berscheid, as discussed in Chapter 1, it does appear that they have taken a back seat to physical beauty. In other words, do not underestimate the importance of how you look. The decade of the 1980's seems greatly influenced by a new wave of people who are interested in body beauty and fitness.

Most people have little control over the social behavior of others. But you can try to understand the reasoning behind some of the behavior, whether you agree with it or not, and intelligently work with it to reach your goals.

Physical Fitness Defined

Q. *Exactly what is physical fitness?*

A. The classical definition of physical fitness centers on an individual's ability to perform his or her daily work with vigor and still have energy left for enjoying hobbies and for meeting unforeseen emergencies.

The above definition is relative, however, because it depends on the occupation, hobbies, and potential emergencies of that person. Obviously, a professional athlete needs a different level of fitness than a career woman. But many career women have special problem areas that merit immediate attention.

Athletic or performance-related fitness usually requires a higher level of commitment than health-related fitness. But regardless of the degree of fitness desired, the basic components are identical. Your body deserves to operate as efficiently as an athlete's.

The basic components of physical fitness are muscular strength, cardiovascular endurance, joint flexibility, and body leanness. Every woman needs a certain amount of these four components in order to function at her best. The required amount is dependent on her genetic potential in each category, as well as her specific needs and desires.

Nautilus Training and Cardiovascular Endurance

Q. *Some people say that Nautilus training works only the skeletal muscles. How does it contribute to cardiovascular endurance?*

A. Nautilus training obviously does promote improvements in muscular strength. But it can also provide high levels of cardiovascular endurance. The key is practicing Nautilus training at the proper pace.

Traditionally, strength training was performed in spurts: 15 to 20 seconds of intense exercise followed by several minutes of rest. Such on-again and off-again lifting might continue for over two hours. Occasionally the trainee's heart rate might be elevated to the necessary level to produce heart-lung endurance, but it quickly returned below the target zone. Usually the particular strength-training exercises were not continued long enough, and more often the rest periods were too long. A trainee might improve muscular strength in this fashion, but little cardiovascular endurance would be produced.

Proper Nautilus training modifies both the duration of the specific exercise and the length of the rest periods. Instead of lifting heavy weights for 15 to 20 seconds, the resistance is reduced and the lifting and lowering of each repetition is performed slowly, smoothly, and rhythmically for approximately 1 minute. Quickly then, within 15 seconds, the trainee moves to the next machine and performs another minute's worth. This continues throughout a maximum of 12 different machines or exercises.

The intensity of the initial Nautilus exercises will effectively raise the woman's heart rate to the upper limits of her target heart-rate zone. During the 10 to 15 seconds that she takes to move from one exercise to the next, her heart rate will decrease to the target zone's lower level. But with the continuation of another exercise, her heart rate will again increase. Thus a reasonably fit woman's heart rate might be elevated to 180 beats per minute for the majority of the 12 exercises, and be no lower than 120 beats per minute during the brief rest periods. Her average heart rate for the entire 15-minute workout would be 150 beats per minute. Such a workout will most definitely improve her cardiovascular endurance.

If the program is properly planned and practiced, every major muscle group in the body can be worked to exhaustion while training the heart and lungs at an optimum level. Individual muscle groups will be worked anaerobically, but the heart and lungs will be worked aerobically. Proper strength training, therefore, has the potential to significantly improve the skeletal muscles and the heart and lungs.

A single program that produces muscular strength and cardiovascular endurance is much more desirable than two separate programs. It is more beneficial to the body as a whole and more successful. It makes fewer demands on the recovery ability and saves time.

Recommended Workout

Q. *What is a recommended Nautilus program for cardiovascular endurance?*

A. Any of the basic routines that are listed in Chapter 13 will contribute to high levels of cardiovascular endurance, if they are performed properly. Remember, for cardiovascular improvements to occur, you must perform each exercise for approximately 60 seconds—and you must move quickly (10 to 15 seconds) from one exercise to the next.

Fun or Torture?

Q. *Many advertisements for fitness centers lead me to believe that exercising is fun. I've also heard that proper exercise is the opposite of fun. What's the truth?*

A. Proper exercise challenges the human body. It acts as a stimulus which forces the body to overcompensate and get stronger. Soon, however, the body adapts to the same stimulus and the stimulus must be made more intense.

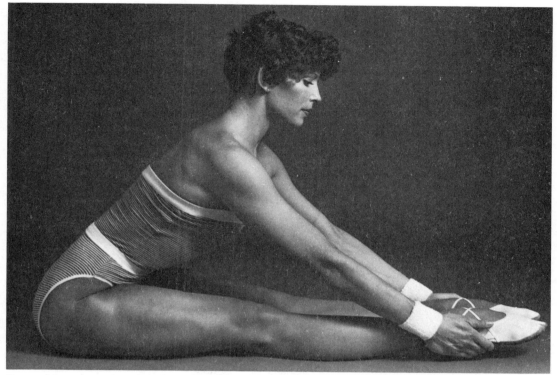

Some of the primary benefits of Nautilus exercise are the strengthening, firming, and shaping that take place throughout the major muscles of the body.

Exercise would only be fun to people who enjoy high levels of physiological stress. The vast majority of people do not enjoy the uncomfortable feelings that occur when muscles are repetitively stretched and contracted and the heart and lungs are forced to provide large amounts of oxygen to the working muscles. When exercise becomes fun, it usually produces only maintenance results.

"It's torture, but it works," is the theme of a very successful fitness center in California. While proper exercise may not be torture, it is certainly rather limited in the fun area.

The fun part of Nautilus exercise comes when you have reached a level of fitness that you are satisfied with. Then you can stay at that level with only maintenance training.

Furthermore, the fun part comes when you see the changes in the mirror and the man you care about notices and compliments you on your looking so slim, strong, and sexy.

Social Aspects

Q. *What about the social aspects of physical fitness?*

A. An interesting study was done recently in Canada to determine why women joined a fitness class. The top three reasons were as follows:

1. To meet new people
2. To socialize
3. To have fun

None of these reasons had anything to do with improving the basic components of fitness. Yet these women were supposedly joining an exercise class. People who desire a more social life should join a country club, not a fitness center. To meet new people, to socialize, and to have fun should be supplemental attractions, rewards for determined effort.

Dancercise

Q. *Dancercise and jazzercise are both advertised as being fun. Is a woman who participates in these wasting her time?*

A. The answer to this question depends on the reason the woman is taking the class. Properly performed dancing movements will contribute to cardiovascular endurance if they elevate the woman's heart to the desired level for an extended period of time. But dance movements will not increase a woman's muscular strength or joint flexibility.

Developing muscular strength requires the body to move through specific ranges of movement against heavy resistance. Dancercise does not effectively isolate the large muscles of the body, nor does it supply the correct resistance to a majority of the appropriate body parts.

Increasing joint flexibility best occurs when a person progressively stretches the major joints of her body in a slow, deliberate manner. Much of the stretching involved in dancing is usually done in a fast, jerky fashion in a nonprogressive manner. Such fast stretching can contribute to loose ligaments which are prone to injury.

Thus, if a woman is interested in improving her muscular strength and joint flexibility, dancercise and jazzercise would be poor choices. Dancing movements would be one way to increase cardiovascular endurance, but even so, it would soon cease to be fun if a woman progressed past a moderate level of endurance.

Misleading Fitness Classes

Q. *Many fitness classes seem to operate under the idea that "something is better than nothing," that almost any type of movement is better than just sitting at home watching television. Is this concept correct?*

A. Arthur Jones, president of Nautilus Sports/Medical Industries, recently addressed the Florida Physical Education Association's annual meeting in Orlando. He estimated that if everyone in the United States realistically rated their physical fitness experiences throughout their lifetime, on a scale from -10 to $+10$, the combined overall average would be -4. In other words, physical fitness activities have caused more harm than good. He also stated that if everyone in the United States suddenly stopped participating in all fitness activities, the health of the nation would significantly improve in a matter of weeks, because their physical fitness experiences would rise from -4 to something closer to 0.

Although the above is an opinion and not a proved fact, national medical records do reveal that each year sport and fitness activities are responsible for 20 million accidents serious enough to require the attention of a doctor. That is more casualties in one year than American troops have suffered in all our wars put together.

The above data reveal that there are serious problems with the physical fitness situation in the United States. Much of this is a result of the proliferation of fitness frauds and easy-exercise methods.

It is unfortunate when "nothing is better than something" may be more appropriate than "something is better than nothing."

Exercise should prevent injury, not cause it. Exercise should improve health, not erode it. And proper exercise performed on Nautilus equipment will accomplish these goals faster and more efficiently than any other form of exercise.

Facts About Muscular Strength

Q. *Exactly what causes muscles to become stronger?*

A. Muscles, which are involved in all human movement, exist in three basic types. The muscles used for body movement are under voluntary, conscious control. These are called skeletal muscles. The heart, automatically operated by the nervous system and not under conscious control, is composed of another kind of tissue called cardiac muscle. A third type of tissue, called smooth muscle, automatically serves internal functions, propelling food through the stomach and intestines and constricting blood vessels to adjust blood flow.

The three types of muscles are all interrelated, but only the voluntary skeletal muscles benefit directly from exercise. Cardiac muscle is strengthened by proper exercise, but this effect is secondary, as a result of increased demand on the circulatory system by the skeletal muscles. Skeletal muscles, therefore, are the key to overall body shape and fitness.

The skeletal muscles are composed of millions of strands of a thin filament protein called actin and a thick filament protein called myosin. Given the presence of calcium, magnesium, and two other proteins called troponin and tropomyosin, actin and myosin can contract and move your limbs with great force.

The fuel for muscular contraction is a chemical compound called adenosine triphosphate, or ATP. When one of the three phosphates has broken off from ATP to form ADP, or adenosine diphosphate, energy is released into the muscular environment. When the actin binds to myosin in the presence of calcium, the energy released from ATP breakdown is used to pull the actin filaments along the myosin filaments. More specifically, a bridge forms between actin and myosin. Energy from ATP breakdown is used to shorten the actomyosin cross-bridge, which shortens the muscle.

When a muscle is contracted repeatedly against resistance, it overcompensates by growing larger and stronger. The technical term for muscular growth is hypertrophy. The signal for hypertrophy is clearly intensity of contraction. When a muscle is faced with high-intensity requirements, it responds with a protective increase in muscular size and strength.

There are a number of physical changes seen with hypertrophy that explain increased muscular size and strength:

- The actin and particularly the myosin protein filaments increase in size.
- The number of actin/myosin units increases.
- The number of blood capillaries within the fiber may increase.
- The amount of connective tissue may increase.

In summary, when a muscle grows larger and stronger, individual muscle fibers primarily increase their volume by adding units of actin and myosin. The total number of muscle fibers, however, remains the same.

Warming Up

Q. *What about warming up before Nautilus?*

A. There is evidence to support the case for warming up as a safeguard against injury. During the warm-up, the cartilages of the knee increase their thickness and provide a better fit for the surfaces of the knee joint. Frictionlike resistance of the muscle cells is reduced by the higher temperature of the body, and the elasticity of the tendons and ligaments is increased. The change to higher temperature not only increases speed of movement and power potential, but also minimizes risk of injury.

A few degrees' rise in temperature of the muscle cells speeds up the production of energy by one-third. These changes in the human mechanism are similar to those that occur in an automobile as it warms up.

Almost any sequence of light calisthenic movements can be used as a general warm-up to precede a Nautilus training session. Suggested movements include head rotation, side bend, trunk twist, squat, and stationary cycling. A minute of each movement should be sufficient. Specific warming up for each body part occurs during the first four repetitions of each Nautilus exercise.

Cooling Down

Q. *After a workout, should I cool down before taking a shower?*

A. Yes. After your last exercise is completed, you can cool down by walking around the workout area, getting a drink of water, and moving your arms in slow circles. Continue these easy movements until your breathing has returned to normal and your heart rate has slowed. This usually takes 5 to 10 minutes.

Q. *Why is cooling down important?*

A. When you exercise vigorously, blood flow increases to your working muscles. If you stop suddenly, there is a tendency for blood to pool in your arms and legs. Since less blood gets back to your heart, you may become lightheaded. But if you keep your arms and legs moving, there is more efficient return of blood to your heart. A cool-down is therefore like a warm-up in reverse. It allows blood flow to your muscles to gradually return to normal.

Nautilus and Young Girls

Q. *Will a Nautilus program be beneficial to a young girl who is 10 years of age?*

A. Yes, Nautilus will benefit a 10-year-old girl if she can fit properly into the machines. The important requisite in using Nautilus is *not* age, but body size. Children under 5 feet in height will have difficulty using most Nautilus machines. Such youngsters will have problems being correctly aligned in some machines and still be able to reach the movement arm. Small girls and boys who want to exercise should be encouraged to use the freehand exercises that are described in Chapter 15. Once they attain a height of 5 feet, they can successfully integrate Nautilus into their fitness programs.

Nautilus and Older Women

Q. *How about women over the age of 65? Should they use Nautilus?*

A. For those over the age of 65, who are in normal health, there is no better exercise than Nautilus. There are a few people in this age group, however, who should be precluded from vigorous Nautilus exercise. Exercise may aggravate the condition of those who have acute arthritis, anemia, tuberculosis, severe kidney or liver diseases, or severe heart problems. In these cases a physician's recommendation should be rigidly adhered to. A complete medical examination should be a prerequisite for anyone over 65 who is interested in Nautilus exercise.

Selecting a Starting Weight

Q. *What's the lightest weight that I can select on a Nautilus machine?*

A. The lightest starting weight on any Nautilus machine is approximately 20 pounds. This 20 pounds includes the top plate and the selector rod that is connected to the chain and goes in the middle of the weights. Each additional plate on the machine weighs 10 pounds.

Using Saddle Plates

Q. *I can perform 13 repetitions with 20 pounds on the double shoulder machine, but I cannot do even 1 with the next highest weight, which is 30 pounds. Do you have any suggestions?*

A. Progression from 20 to 30 pounds in one jump on any Nautilus machine will be impossible for most women. That is a 50 percent weight progression as opposed to the ideal, which should be 5 percent. Nautilus is now manufacturing small 1¼-, 2½-, 5-, and 7½-pound saddle plates that fit over the top weights on all machines (see pages 32-33). This problem can also be solved by pinning light barbell plates onto the weight stack. By using small weight increments, you will be able to progress in training in a more systematic manner.

Negative Training

Q. *Negative chins and negative dips have been previously described and illustrated. I'd like to know more about performing negative exercise on Nautilus machines.*

A. When you lift the weight stack that is connected to the movement arm of any Nautilus machine, the involved muscles are contracting concentrically and positive work is accomplished. When you lower the weight stack on any Nautilus machine, your muscles are contracting eccentrically, and negative work is performed. Positive work is lifting. Negative work is lowering.

Nautilus research has shown that concentrating on the negative phase of a repetition produces better strengthening and shaping results than emphasizing the positive phase.

That is why it is recommended on a normal repetition that you take twice as long to lower the weight as it takes you to lift it. The guideline is to lift the resistance in 2 seconds and lower it in 4 seconds.

Negative chins and dips on the multi-exercise machine allow you to carry the negative concept even further. Since you can lower more weight than you can lift, it follows that the intensity of the exercise would be higher if you could figure out a way to practice heavy lowering repetitions. The problem, however, is how can you lower a weight you cannot lift? This dilemma has been effectively solved with the multi-exercise machine. You simply lift the weight (your body weight in this case) with your legs and lower it with your arms and torso. This is possible because your legs are several times stronger than your arms and torso. Thus, you can use the strength of your lower body to allow you to work your upper body in the most productive manner.

Any woman who has performed negative chins and dips can testify to the fact that they are two of the very best exercises for the upper body. Most women who are not strong enough to perform a normal positive chin or dip, can improve this specific strength through the use of negative exercise.

An important guideline to remember in doing negative chins and dips is to climb to the top position quickly, but perform the lowering phase very slowly. On your first several repetitions, take 8 to 10 seconds to lower yourself. If this is not possible, have someone grasp your feet and assist you by lifting up on them. When you can no longer control your lowering speed, the exercise should be terminated.

Q. *Are there other ways to emphasize the negative part of Nautilus exercises?*

A. Yes, a popular way to emphasize the negative on some Nautilus machines is called *negative-accentuated training*. For negative-accentuated training the Nautilus machine must have a single-connected movement arm. For example, single-connected movement arms are found on the leg extension, leg curl, pullover, overhead press, and decline press. The idea is to lift the movement arm with both legs or arms and lower it with only one limb.

The leg curl machines offers a good example of negative-accentuated exercise. If you can normally handle 50 pounds for 10 repetitions, you should use 35 pounds. In other words, use 70 percent of the weight you would normally use.

Lift the movement arm with both legs. Pause in the contracted position and smoothly transfer the resistance from both legs to the right leg. Slowly lower the right leg in about 8 seconds. Lift the weight back to the top position with both legs, pause, and lower again, this time with the left leg, in a slow, even manner. Up with two legs, down with one; up with two legs again, down with the other. You should continue until you can no longer raise the weight to the contracted position.

If the weight is selected correctly, you should reach a point of momentary failure at about the eleventh or twelfth lifting repetition. When you can perform 12 repetitions, you should increase the resistance by 5 percent. A properly performed set of negative-accentuated exercise will consist of 8 to 12 lifting movements, plus 4 to 6 negative movements performed by the right leg and an equal number by the left.

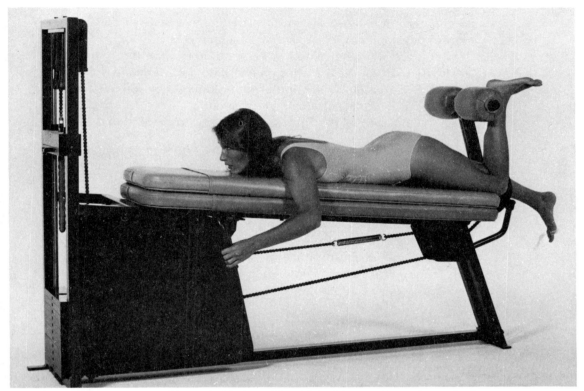

To perform negative-accentuated leg curls, lift the weight with both legs and lower it very slowly with only one leg.

While negative-accentuated exercise is certainly a productive way to train, it should not be attempted until a woman has trained regularly on Nautilus equipment for at least six months. A woman should first double the strength in all her major muscle groups before she attempts negative-accentuated exercise.

More Is Not Better

Q. *I'd like to train on Nautilus more than three times weekly. How should I plan my schedule?*

A. You should realize that when it comes to Nautilus exercise, *more is not better.* It is the quality, not the quantity of the exercise that counts. Proper exercise simply stimulates your body to become stronger. The actual strengthening takes place 24 to 48 hours after the stimulation has occurred. The day-after recovery period is as important as the exercise itself. If you exercise intensely for two or three days in a row, your body will not have sufficient time to recover. The results of such an exercise program will be slow at best and counterproductive at worst. Overtraining is a state of debilitation, not development.

If you are still determined to exercise more than three times weekly, try to make the activities on alternate days light and of low intensity. For example, a 10-minute warm-up might be followed by 15 minutes of moderate stretching movements.

Q. *What about all the successful college and professional athletes who train daily, or even twice daily?*

A. Most college and professional athletes are products of favorable genetics. They are strong and fast primarily because of gifted ancestors. Most successful athletes are undertrained in intensity and overtrained in amount. They are successful in spite of their conditioning programs, rather than because of them.

Perhaps in the future all athletes and fitness-minded people will understand that really productive exercise must be intense and brief. Training twice a day is not better than training once a day. And training every day is not better than training every other day. High-intensity Nautilus exercise as described in this book should be followed by at least a 48-hour recovery period.

Splitting the Workout

Q. *What about performing exercise for the lower body one day and exercise for the upper body the next day? Is this better than training the entire body every other day.*

A. No! The human body functions best by working all the major muscle groups in close proximity to one another. Splitting the workouts into upper body one day and lower body the next makes about as much sense as eating or sleeping for one part of the body. The body functions best when it is worked in its entirety and then is allowed to rest in its entirety.

Muscles Turning to Fat

Q. *What happens if a woman strength-trains and gets into good condition and then stops working out? Will her muscles turn to fat?*

A. Absolutely not! Muscles are muscles, and fat is fat. There is no way a woman can turn one into the other.

Muscles are composed of 70 percent water, 22 percent proteins, and 7 percent lipids. Fat is 22 percent water, 6 percent protein, and 72 percent lipids. So, like apples and oranges, muscle and fat, though similar in composition, are genetically and chemically different.

When a conditioned individual stops training, she seldom decreases her caloric intake. As a result, she has a gradual decrease in the shape and strength of her muscle mass and an increase in body fat stores. Since muscle and fat are so close to each other that they can intermingle, it appears that her muscles have turned to fat. Fortunately, this does not happen immediately. She can stop exercising completely and work back to her previous level of condition in a fraction of the time it took in the beginning.

Saddlebags Around the Thighs

Q. *Are there any specific exercises to combat the saddlebags that many women get around the tops of their thighs?*

A. If the saddlebags are caused by excessive fatty deposits, there is little a woman can do without proper dieting. Remember, spot reducing of fatty deposits is impossible. If, however, they are caused partly or entirely by flaccid, out-of-shape muscles, the Nautilus hip and thigh machines will prove helpful.

Cellulite

Q. *The comment about cellulite in Chapter 2 is confusing. Why isn't it a special type of fat that is very difficult to remove?*

A. There is nothing special about cellulite. It's just plain fat. A bit more explanation should help.

The relationship between the skin, the fat, and the underlying muscles are rather distinctive in human beings. Other species have fur, feathers, and certain blood-shunting devices in their bag of cold-weather tricks. But we humans have virtually nothing between us and the elements except fat and skin. This may be one of the reasons that fat adheres so stubbornly to our underlying tissues.

It is this adhesiveness that accounts for the kind of dimpling effect that has been dubbed cellulite. The term has been applied to the puckering or dimpling of fat that occurs in the buttocks and thighs of overfat and usually middle-aged women. Cellulite has become such a common word that it would be pointless to try to remove it from our vocabulary. Although there is no such word medically, the condition to which it refers is one that can and does exist.

What apparently happens in cellulite is that the ribbons of connective tissue, which serve as pouches for large groups of fat cells in a sort of honeycomb arrangement under the skin, lose their elasticity and shrink with age. The overlying skin which is attached to these fibers then contracts. If the size of the fat cells encased in them does not shrink to match, a kind of overall dimpling occurs on the surface of the skin.

Another contributing factor to the problem is that most women after the age of 18 years gradually lose muscular size and strength in their hips and thighs. This reduction in strength makes the underlying muscle mass flabbier and less supportive of the surrounding fat and skin.

Q. *Is there a cure for the cellulite look?*

A. The cure for cellulite, or dimpled fatty deposits, is a two-fold approach:

1. You must reduce the size of the enpouched fat by dieting. A well-balanced, low-calorie diet (from 1,200 to 1,500 calories a day) is the recommended way to reduce the enpouched fat.

2. You must increase the size and strength of the large muscles that compose the hips and thighs. The other major muscles should also be exercised to support fatty deposits throughout the body. The most efficient form of exercise is performed on Nautilus equipment.

Massage

Q. *It feels good to massage my fat bulges. Does massage help to flush out fat?*

A. Massaging those fatty deposits on your thighs and hips may feel good, but it will not break down and flush out the components of fat cells. It is impossible to knead, knuckle, wring, shake, beat, or stroke fat from the human body.

Body Wraps

Q. *Recently, I've read about a method called a body wrap that supposedly helps to dissolve cellulite and tighten the skin. What is a body wrap?*

A. One popular method of body wrapping is as follows:

1. Circumference measurements in inches are taken on various parts of a woman's body.

2. Elastic bandages that have been soaked in warm, distilled water with "secret minerals and additives" are then wound tightly around the woman's entire body from the ankles up and to the neck and hands.

3. After the wrapping is complete, the woman puts on a baggy plastic jacket and pants. Plastic bags are also put on her feet.

4. The woman is then led to a warm room where she is instructed to sit and relax for 60 to 90 minutes.

5. After 60 to 90 minutes, the plastic-encased woman is taken back to the first room where she is unwrapped and quickly re-measured.

6. The woman then receives a record of the inch differences, but not the before and after measurements. Advertisements claim that most women lose 6 to 8 inches during the first wrap. She is instructed not to bathe for 14 to 16 hours because she can lose more inches by leaving the solution on longer.

7. The cost of body wrap is usually from $25 to $50 for each treatment.

Other types of body wraps include rubbing various creams on the body's fat areas and covering them with Saran wrap. Sometimes the wrapped woman is encouraged to do calisthenic-type exercises instead of sitting. Another technique even hooks a vacuum cleaner to the woman's plastic pants. This method supposedly "sucks fat away!"

Q. *Is the body wrap effective in dissolving cellulite and tightening the skin?*

A. No! If there was a strong chemical that would actually dissolve fat, it would also dissolve your skin, muscles, and other components of your body as well.

Body wrapping, one of the latest fads to remove fat, involves covering the body with elastic bandages that have been soaked in a saline solution. Such wrapping may temporarily compact a body part, but it does nothing to shrink the underlying fat cells.

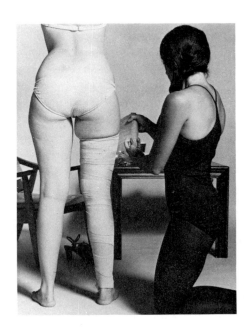

As for a body wrap tightening the skin, this is also impossible. Elasticity of the skin is primarily determined by the condition of the skin's collagen fibers. Collagen fibers are not influenced by rubbing a cream or solution on the surface of the skin. What apparently gives a wrapped person the feeling that her skin is tightening is the fact that the cream or the solution that the wraps have been soaked in contains a bit of menthol, wintergreen, or cinnamon oil. These substances provide a warming-cooling sensation when they are rubbed onto the body. This would not tighten or shrink the skin, however.

Q. *If body wraps do not work, how do the before and after measurements show an average loss of 6 to 8 inches?*

A. There are three ways this could happen, and all of them are temporary at best.

First, by wrapping the body tightly you are compacting the tissues, or squeezing fluids up or down. This is easily observed when you wear a pair of nylon socks with a tight elastic band to hold them in place. Wear the socks for an hour, then take them off and you will observe an indentation where the elastic band was. The identation goes away in a matter of minutes as the fluids return to the area.

Second, body wraps and plastic suits can cause perspiration. Excessive perspiration can lead to dehydration. This could produce serious overheating problems, especially if the woman tries to exercise vigorously or sits in a sauna. Excessive sweating actually causes your body to preserve its fat stores, not to use them. Furthermore, any inches lost through dehydration would return as soon as you quenched your thirst.

Third, circumference measurements of the body are very easy to manipulate. Take three separate measurements, 30 seconds apart, around the top of the thigh and all three may vary. By pulling the tape measure tighter, by slightly moving higher or lower on the body part, by taking the before measurements at an angle, or by simply fudging on the data, a clever technician can make a woman believe that many inches are being lost from her body. This is especially true when 15 to 30 separate measurements are taken. In fact, the more measurements the better, because this increases the possibility of having more differences and more inches.

Fat Distribution

Q. *Why do most women store the majority of their fat on their hips and thighs?*

A. Before puberty, girls have only slightly more fat than boys. At the end of adolescence, they have twice as much fat as boys. Some scientists think this additional fat is programmed into the potential mother's body to insure the species' continuity. Thus, the primary reason that women store over twice as much fat on their hips and thighs as do men may be directly related to the female's potential for pregnancy and motherhood.

Sports-medicine scientists have noted that lean women athletes may have difficulty becoming pregnant. Evidently, when a woman's body fat gets below approximately 10 percent of her body weight, her hormone levels are decreased. This usually affects ovulation and menstruation. A lean woman may have to gain body fat in order to get pregnant.

Not only does additional fat contribute to conception, but it also offers protection to the woman's vital organs and her unborn fetus. Fat also provides a built-in energy source so the mother and child can survive at least for a while on the mother's stored fat.

It seems that one of the unique physical characteristics of women, the ability to conceive children, also is a key to why women store large amounts of fat on their hips and thighs.

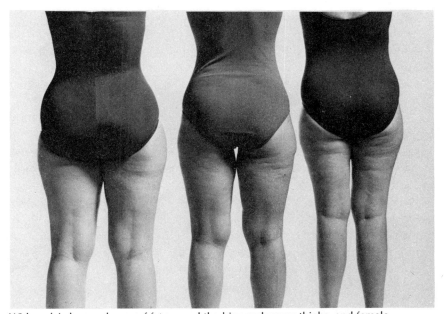

Wide pelvic bones, layers of fat around the hips and upper thighs, and female hormones are evolutionary factors that give women the potential to conceive and bear children. These three factors, combined with the natural aging process and a lack of proper exercise, often lead to the condition in the above picture. This condition can be improved by a low-calorie diet to shrink the fat cells and a Nautilus exercise program to strengthen the supporting muscles.

Sagging Breasts

Q. *Will proper exercise keep a woman's breasts from sagging?*

A. Large breasts, and even medium-sized breasts, are going to sag eventually from the aging process that naturally occurs. As a woman gradually ages, the elasticity is slowly reduced in her connective tissue, ligaments, and skin. Of course, keeping the supporting muscles underneath and surrounding the breasts as strong as possible will help to maintain a firm bustline.

Double Chin

Q. *Is there any special exercise that will eliminate a double chin?*

A. There are no exercises that will eliminate the fat from under the chin or that will change how a person stores fat. The mechanical vibrating straps that are frequently seen in health spas are totally unproductive. Once again, spot reducing is an outright myth.

The best thing for a woman with a double chin to do is to reduce her overall body fat, and strengthen the muscles of her neck through the use of the Nautilus 4-way neck machine.

Reaching Fatigue

Q. *In performing on a specific Nautilus machine, how do I know when my muscles have reached the point of fatigue?*

A. All exercises on Nautilus machines should be performed throughout a full range of motion—smoothly and slowly without sudden, jerky movements. Assuming this rule is closely followed, movements are continued until proper execution becomes impossible. At this point fatigue is reached. Most people will experience a burning sensation several repetitions preceding fatigue in a given exercise. This sensation is normal and should be tolerated to obtain best results.

As you become stronger and shapelier, the exercises will become progressively more strenuous. If they do not become more strenuous, you are wasting much of your effort.

Keeping Accurate Records

Q. *How do I measure the progress of my Nautilus program?*

A. The best way to measure progress is by keeping accurate records of all your workouts (see Nautilus Training Record on page 146). You should have a fitness diary to record such things as:

1. Date
2. Time of day
3. Listing of exercises
4. Amount of resistance
5. Number of correct repetitions
6. Total workout time

If you perform 10 repetitions of an exercise on Monday, you can set your sights for 11 or 12 on the following Wednesday. Keeping track of your progress can help to challenge and encourage you to continue and to set appropriate goals.

Photographs can be used to provide a visual record of your progress. During the beginning stages of your Nautilus program, put on your bathing suit and have full-length photographs taken against an uncluttered background. Don't try to pose or flex your muscles. Stand perfectly relaxed for three pictures: front, side, and back. Repeat the picture-taking sessions every two months. Compare the photographs with the preceding sets. Before-and-after pictures are excellent reminders of your past and present states of fatness and fitness.

Combining Running and Nautilus

Q. *What is the best way to combine running with Nautilus?*

A. The best way is to do both activities on the same day. Under ideal conditions, the trainee would run in the morning and train on Nautilus in the afternoon. There should be approximately four hours' time lapse between both activities, with a complete day's rest afterward. An every-other-day schedule like this produces the best combined results.

Most people, however, because of the inconvenience of training twice in one day, would rather run on one day, and perform Nautilus the next. Or they will try to do both activities on the same day with only a brief rest in between. Neither of these methods has proved to be superior in results to the first combination program.

Sickness and Exercise

Q. *Should a fitness-minded woman try to exercise when she is feeling sick?*

A. No! A woman should not try to exercise when she is sick. Both exercise and illness make heavy demands on an individual's recovery ability. A woman's recovery ability does not increase in proportion to her ability to gain strength.

Sickness and infections require maximum degrees of recovery ability. Continuing to exercise during periods of illness retards the trainee's ability to recover. It can actually aggravate the illness.

As a rule, a woman should rest one day for every day she was sick before resuming her Nautilus program. When she starts again, she should exercise at a lower intensity for several days.

Be sure, however, that the word "sick" is never used to replace "lazy," "apathetic," or "hypochondriacal." Sick is not synonymous with these terms. There are many excuses for avoiding exercise. There are many more reasons to accept the challenge and reap its benefits.

Higher Repetitions

Q. *Will a woman get better bodyshaping results if she performs more than 12 repetitions on some Nautilus machines?*

A. Repetitions are not as important as time. Skeletal muscle strength is produced by working with the anaerobic metabolic processes. The anaerobic metabolic processes are best taxed by intensive, continuous exercise that lasts at least 30 seconds, but not more than 70 seconds. Continuing an exercise past 70 seconds may involve the aerobic processes, or heart and lungs, to a greater degree than the skeletal muscles. A repetition correctly performed on a Nautilus machine, depending on the range of movement, takes from 3 to 8 seconds. If a typical repetition takes about 6 seconds to perform, simple multiplication reveals that 8 repetitions would equal 48 seconds, and 12 repetitions would equal 72 seconds.

Eight to 12 repetitions, or 30 to 70 seconds, apply to almost all Nautilus machines. The two major exceptions are the duo hip and back and duo squat machines, which are performed by alternating legs. In the duo hip and back and duo squat machines, as one leg is performing the complete range of movement, the other leg is locked out or holding static in the contracted position. In other words, the exercise is *not* performed continuously for both legs together. One leg is always recovering somewhat as the other leg is working. Depending on the degree of recovery that takes place between each repetition, you might be able to perform 20 repetitions or more with each leg on the duo hip and back and duo squat machines. This is particularly true with the squat machine. You might have to stay on the duo squat machine for 2½ to 3 minutes before you thoroughly fatigue the involved muscles of both legs.

Generally speaking, 8 to 12 repetitions is the best guideline to follow on the other Nautilus machines. Use 15 to 20 repetitions on the duo hip and back and duo squat, which are performed by alternating legs. If Nautilus makes a version of the hip and back and squat machines that can be done with both legs together, 8 to 12 repetitions would be sufficient.

Training Expectations

Q. *What can an average woman expect from strict adherence to a Nautilus program for six months?*

A. The average woman who trains on Nautilus consistently for six months can expect to double her strength in all her major muscle groups. If on January 1, she performs 30 pounds for 10 repetitions on the leg extension machine, then by July 1, if she has trained progressively, she should be able to perform 60 pounds for 10 repetitions. Since the leg extension works the quadriceps muscles, her quadriceps are twice as strong. The same increases would apply to the major muscles that are worked by the other Nautilus machines.

Since 1970, many women have trained at the Nautilus Research Center in Lake Helen, Florida. A large majority of them have doubled their strength in six months. A few have tripled their strength in some muscle groups.

Doubling your strength significantly improves your entire body. Your inside body will be leaner, stronger, more flexible, and more enduring. Your outside body will be sleeker, shapelier, and firmer. And those problem areas that you may have, such as flabby hips and thighs, or skinny arms and calves, can be selectively toned and contoured to make your overall appearance more symmetrical.

And what effect does doubling or even tripling a woman's strength have on her overall lifestyle? The effects will vary depending on the woman's occupation, habits, age, and many other lifestyle factors. But in all activities that involve muscular movement, such as walking, running, driving, lifting, carrying, pushing, pulling, and thousands of other actions, there will be a vast improvement in efficiency. Furthermore, she will be more resistant to injury.

Side Leg Curl

Q. *What's the reason behind the side leg curl machine?*

A. The side leg curl was originally designed so a pregnant woman could conveniently and comfortably exercise her hamstrings. By lying on her side to perform the leg curl, minimum compression forces are exerted on her front abdominal area.

After testing the machine with many pregnant women, however, we discovered that other women and men also enjoyed using the side leg curl. If you have access to both machines, you may use either in your regular workouts. Or you may alternate between the leg curl and the side leg curl. Both work your hamstrings in a progressive manner.

Nautilus Home Machines

Q. *What's the latest on the Nautilus home machines?*

A. Nautilus home machines are lightweight versions of the heavy-duty commercial machines. The home machines do not have steel weight stacks. The various resistance settings are possible through the use of specially designed rubberized cords. Available home machines include the abdominal, lower back, hip and back, biceps, triceps, stationary cycles, and a treadmill. The home abdominal and lower back are detailed below.

Home Abdominal Machine

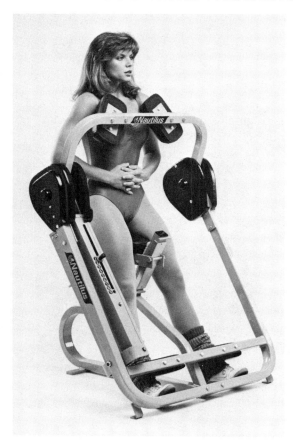

1. Sit in machine with swivel pads in front of chest.
2. Adjust seat until axis of rotation of movement arm is parallel to navel.
3. Hook feet under bottom foot pads.
4. Adjust swivel pads on chest to comfortable position.
5. Place hands across waist.
6. Keep knees wide.

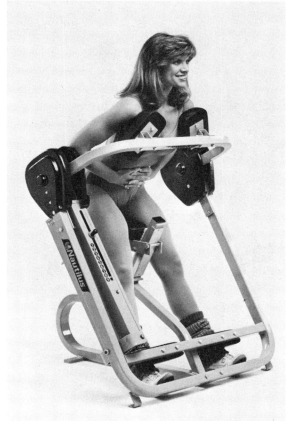

7. Crunch torso downward toward seat bottom.
8. Pause in contracted position.
9. Return slowly to starting position.
10. Repeat.

Home Lower Back Machine

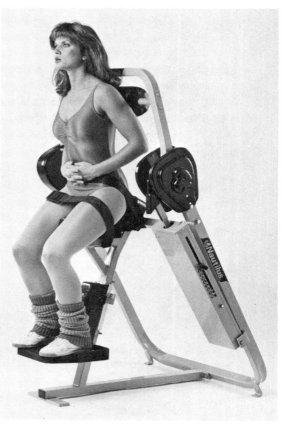

1. Sit on seat bottom with feet on foot rest.
2. Adjust foot rest until knees are slightly bent and lower back is positioned on same level as axis of rotation of machine.
3. Secure belts tightly, first across thighs and then across hips.
4. Stabilize feet, interlace hands across waist, and place upper back against top roller pad.

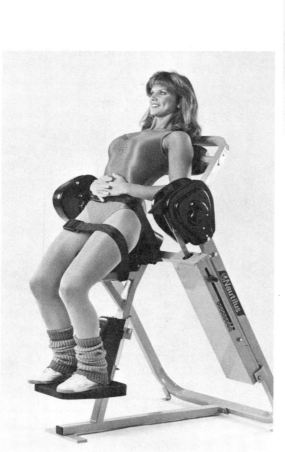

5. Press smoothly against roller pad and move torso back until in line with thighs.
6. Pause in rear position. Do not arch back excessively.
7. Bend forward slowly to starting position. Keep upper back straight at all times. Do not round over.
8. Repeat as many repetitions as possible in good form.

Nautilus Diet Program

Q. *Is there a recommended low-calorie diet to combine with Nautilus training for efficient fat loss?*

A. Yes, I have written a new book, *The Nautilus Diet,* for this purpose. The book presents a unique 10-week program of low-calorie eating combined with Nautilus exercise. Each 2-week period requires you to reduce your calories and increase the intensity of your exercise. By following this program consistently for 10 weeks, the average overfat woman can expect to lose 20 pounds of fat, trim 6 inches off her hips and thighs, and increase both her upper and lower body strength by at least 25 percent.

For further information on *The Nautilus Diet,* please send a self-addressed, stamped envelope to Darden Research Corporation, P.O. Box 1016, Lake Helen FL 32744.

Using Nautilus When Pregnant

Q. *I've been using Nautilus for almost a year. Several days ago I learned that I'm two months pregnant. Should I keep training on Nautilus?*

A. Generally speaking, yes. If you are having an uncomplicated pregnancy, the prenatal period of your life need not be a period of passivity. In fact, just the opposite should be true.

Giving birth involves the relaxation and contraction of many major muscle groups, such as the uterus, abdominals, gluteals, quadriceps, adductors, and hamstrings. If these muscles are strong and flexible, you should have an easier time at birth. Also, you will feel and look better—before and after the baby is born.

Dr. Douglas C. Hall, an obstetrician in Ocala, Florida, has personally supervised over 600 pregnant women on Nautilus equipment. He has found that, compared to pregnant women who do not practice high-intensity exercise, the Nautilus-trained women had significantly fewer:

1. Orthopedic problems
2. Gynecological complications
3. Labor contractions
4. Birth difficulties
5. Caesarian sections

Dr. Hall does point out, however, that there are a few pregnant women with certain medical problems who should *not* do Nautilus or any other strenuous exercise. Plus, it should be noted that a pregnant woman's physical fitness does not always guarantee easy labor, delivery and recuperation. If you are pregnant, or planning to become pregnant, be sure to make your obstetrician thoroughly aware of your exercise habits and adhere to your doctor's recommendations.

Q. *Are there Nautilus machines that a pregnant woman should not use?*

A. The Nautilus machines that are performed lying on the back could cause complications. The duo hip and back machine, the hip flexion machine, and the 10° chest machine fall into this category. When a pregnant woman is positioned in these machines, there is a possibility that the enlarging uterus will compress the inferior vena cava. Compression of the inferior vena cava may result in reduced blood pressure and a decrease in the heart rate of the fetus. What effect this has on the fetus will depend on the state of the pregnancy and how long the woman is in the supine position. Unless you are being monitored in your Nautilus training by an obstetrician, it is best to forego the duo hip and back, hip flexion, and 10° chest machines during the last several months of pregnancy.

In place of the two hip machines, a pregnant woman could substitute the Nautilus duo squat machine. The angle of the back pad on the duo squat seems to eliminate compression on the inferior vena cava. Instead of the 10° chest, a woman could use the women's chest or arm cross.

A pregnant woman should also be careful of the hip adduction machine during the last trimester. Too much stretching in the groin area, combined with increasing hormone levels, can cause the adductor muscles to pull away from the hip bones.

The enlarging uterus will gradually preclude a pregnant woman from using the leg curl and abdominal machines. The side leg curl and the pullover may be substituted. All other Nautilus machines can be used with regularity throughout a normal, healthy pregnancy.

Stretch Marks

Q. *Does every pregnant woman get stretch marks? What can I do about them?*

A. Stretch marks, which often appear on the breasts and abdomen during pregnancy, are due to the tearing of elastic tissues in the skin that accompanies enlargement of the breasts, distention of the abdomen, and deposition of subcutaneous fat. They are pink or purplish-red lines on the skin during pregnancy. The lines become permanent grayish-white, scarlike marks after delivery. Some women never develop stretch marks despite bearing several children; others can lose skin tone after one pregnancy. Evidently there is an inherited factor involved. Stretch marks cannot be considered evidence that a woman has borne a child, however, because they are seen on women who have not been pregnant.

Once stretch marks appear there is nothing to be done about them. You can help to prevent them, however, by being sure you do not gain excessive amounts of body fat, by adhering to a well-balanced diet, and by keeping your muscles in good condition.

Varicose Veins and Pregnancy

Q. *How are varicose veins related to pregnancy?*

A. Varicose veins are bulging, twisted, and knotted veins that are usually located right under the skin. While they frequently occur in pregnant women, they appear in other women and men as well. Most often they develop in the legs, although they can pop out in other places like the anal area (hemorrhoids) and the genital area. Their presence is due to two factors. One, many pregnancies contribute to a generally weakened condition of the veins in the legs if the pressure created by the baby cuts off some of the circulation. Two, a tendency toward varicose veins can be genetic. In such a case, the individual probably inherited a tendency toward inelasticity in the vein walls.

In both instances, however, the results are the same: There is a weakness or malfunction within the flaplike valves of the vein. As the weight of the blood on the vein wall increases, the vein bulges, and after long stretching, it loses its elasticity and finally becomes elongated, twisted, and knotted.

Preventing Varicose Veins

Q. *Will Nautilus exercise help varicose veins?*

A. Yes. Any type of contracting or pumping of the leg muscles helps to milk the blood out of the calves and propel it upward toward the heart. Brisk walking helps, but calf raises and squats are even better. Everyone can benefit by maintaining strength in the thigh and calf muscles. The strong, firm muscles around deep veins help provide external support and protection from overstretching and damage.

Q. *Can varicose veins be prevented?*

A. If you have a genetic predisposition for varicose veins, you probably will not be able to prevent them. These measures, however, will help to minimize them:

- Avoid standing for long periods. If you must stand, wear lightweight support stockings. When standing on the bus, at your job, or at the kitchen sink, flex your toes every few minutes and then rise slowly on your tiptoes.
- Do not sit for long periods, especially with your legs crossed. When sitting, elevate your legs or change their position. On long train, plane, or bus trips, walk about every half hour. On long car trips, switch drivers frequently or stop for light exercise every hour, if possible.
- Avoid tight garments that constrict your legs: girdles, garters, and knee-high stockings. High boots with elastic around the tops are especially bad.
- Keep your body fat within a normal range.

Miss Nautilus Contest

Q. *I read last spring that Nautilus Sports/Medical Industries sponsored a Miss Nautilus Contest. How was it judged, who won, and will there be other contests?*

A. Yes, the Miss Nautilus Contest was held at Arthur and Terri Jones's JumboLair Ranch in Ocala, Florida. Two separate contests were held: one for Florida residents and the other for Georgia residents. Twenty finalists from each state were selected from several hundred entries.

The contest was judged on four factors: (1) personal interview, (2) modeling ability in a one-piece bathing suit, (3) modeling ability in a bikini, and (4) general appearance, which included hair, skin, face, figure, and poise. A cash prize of $5,000 was awarded to each winner.

The two winners were Lori Brown of Orlando, Florida, and Sharon Smith of Marietta, Georgia.

A National Miss Nautilus Contest is planned for the summer of 1986 and annually thereafter. For further information, please write: Miss Nautilus Contest, Nautilus Sports/Medical Industries, P. O. Box 1783, DeLand, FL 32720.

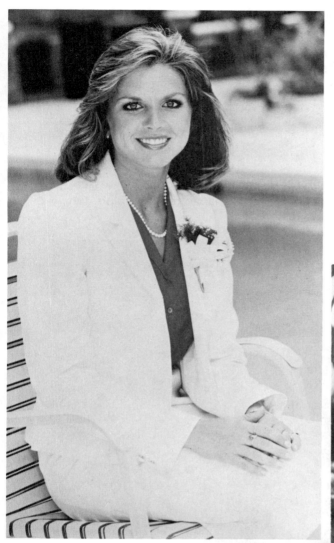

Lori Brown of Orlando, Florida.

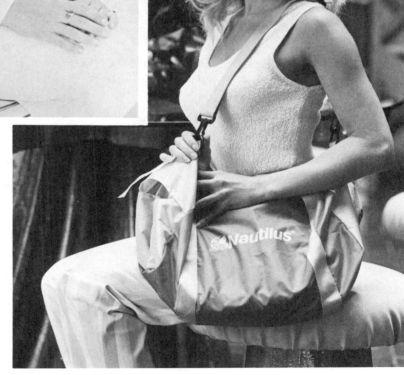

Sharon Smith of Marietta, Georgia.

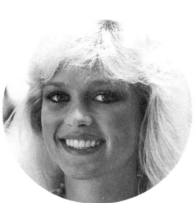

Tasha Auer

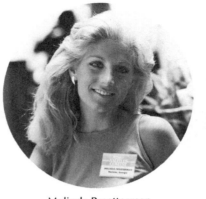

Melinda Prostterman

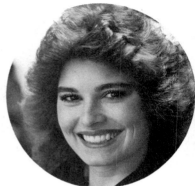

Diana Lynch

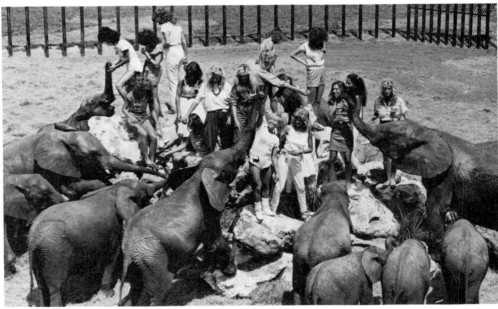

A group of Miss Nautilus contestants feed and enjoy the attention of some of the 85 baby elephants, which are housed at the JumboLair Ranch in Ocala, Florida. The JumboLair added an interesting background for the contestants, some of which are pictured on this page.

Hope Marie

Patricia Lynn Binette

Debra Burnsworth

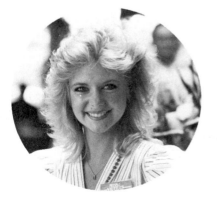

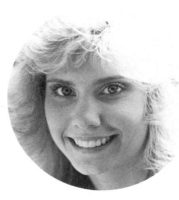

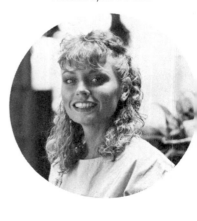

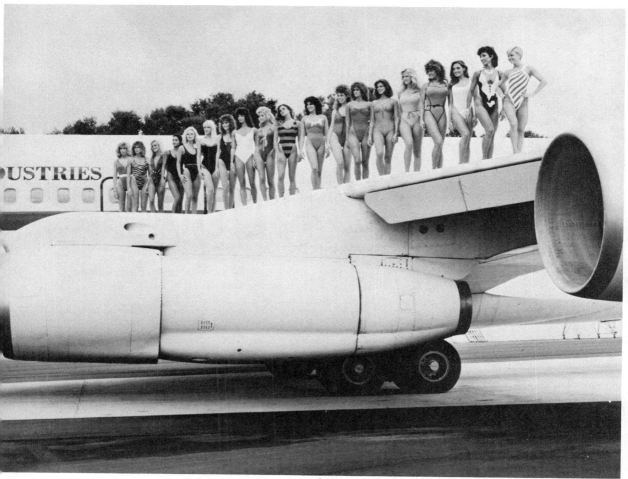

A partial line-up of Miss Nautilus finalists on the wing of one of the Nautilus 707 Jumbo Jets.

This should answer the questions that have been puzzling you about Nautilus. You should be ready now to start your Nautilus program and attain the fit, attractive body that you have always wanted.

Conclusion

Nautilus exercise will make you slimmer, stronger, sexier, and simultaneously improve your health. When you feel healthy and look attractive, you will have poise and confidence. You will be an alluring, vibrant person.

If you consistently follow the guidelines presented in this book, your results will certainly exceed your highest expectations.

Expect a lot. You are a Nautilus woman!

Bibliography

Barrett, Stephen, ed. *The Health Robbers.* Philadelphia: George F. Stickley, Publishers, 1980.

Beller, Anne Scott. *Fat and Thin.* New York: Farrar, Straus and Giroux, 1977.

Berscheid, Ellen, and Walster, Elaine. "Beauty and the Best." *Psychology Today* 5:42–46, 74, March 1972.

Berscheid, Ellen. "Physical Attractiveness." In *Advances in Experimental Social Psychology,* ed. L. Berkowitz, 7:157–215, 1974.

———."An Overview of the Psychological Effects of Physical Attractiveness." In *Psychological Aspects of Facial Form,* eds. G. W. Lucker, K. A. Ribbens, and J. A. McNamara. Ann Arbor, Michigan: Center for Human Growth and Development, 1981.

Brown, C., and Wilmore, Jack. "The Effects of Maximal Resistance Training on the Strength and Body Composition of Women Athletes." *Medicine and Science in Sports* 6:174–77, 1974.

Darden, Ellington. *The Nautilus Nutrition Book.* Chicago: Contemporary Books, Inc., 1981.

———. *The Nautilus Book.* rev. ed. Chicago: Contemporary Books, Inc., 1985.

———. *The Nautilus Bodybuilding Book.* rev. ed. Chicago: Contemporary Books, Inc., 1986.

———. *The Darden Technique for Weight Loss, Body Shaping and Slenderizing.* New York: Simon & Schuster, 1982.

Fox, Edward L., and Mathews, Donald K. "Chapter 14. Exercise and Training in Females." *The Physiological Basis of Physical Education and Athletes.* 3d ed. Philadelphia: Saunders College Publishing, 1981.

Freud, Sigmund. *Autobiography.* New York: W. W. Norton & Company, 1935.

Jones, Arthur. *Nautilus Training Principles, Bulletin No. 1.* DeLand, Florida: Nautilus Sports/Medical Industries, 1970.

———. "Nautilus Exercise Guide." *Shape* 1:22–31, May 1982.

Jones, Terri. "Women and Fitness." *Nautilus Magazine* 4:64–65, October–November 1982.

Kendall, H. O.; Kendall, F. P.,; and Wadsworth, G. E. *Muscles: Testing and Function.* Baltimore: Williams & Williams, 1971.

Laubach, L. "Comparative Muscular Strength of Men and Women: A Review of the Literature." *Aviation Space Environmental Medicine* 47:534–42, 1976.

Mathes, Eugene W. "The Effects of Physical Attractiveness and Anxiety on Heterosexual Attraction Over a Series of Five Encounters." *Journal of Marriage and the Family* 769–73, November 1975.

Peterson, James A., ed. *Total Fitness: The Nautilus Way.* 2d ed. West Point, New York: Leisure Press, 1982.

"This Is What You Thought About the Impact of Beauty." *Glamour* 80: 34, April 1982.

Wilmore, Jack. "Body Composition and Strength Development." *Journal of Physical Education and Recreation* 46: 38–40, 1975.

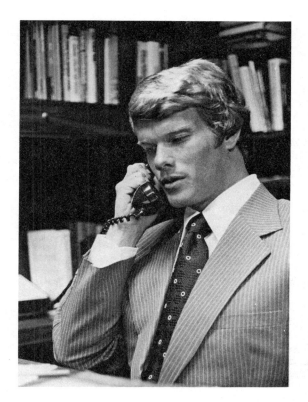

About the Author

Dr. Ellington Darden is an authority in the fields of physical fitness, bodyshaping, and nutrition. He holds B.S. and M.S. degrees from Baylor University, a Ph.D. in physical education from Florida State University, and has had two years of post-doctoral study in food and nutrition. He is a well-known writer and speaker whose books, articles, and lectures are bringing a new awareness of body fitness to Americans of all ages.

As Director of Research for Nautilus Sports/Medical Industries, Dr. Darden has authored numerous training manuals, such as *The Nautilus Book*, *The Nautilus Bodybuilding Book*, *The Nautilus Nutrition Book*, and *How to Lose Body Fat*. *The Nautilus Woman* is his twenty-second book.

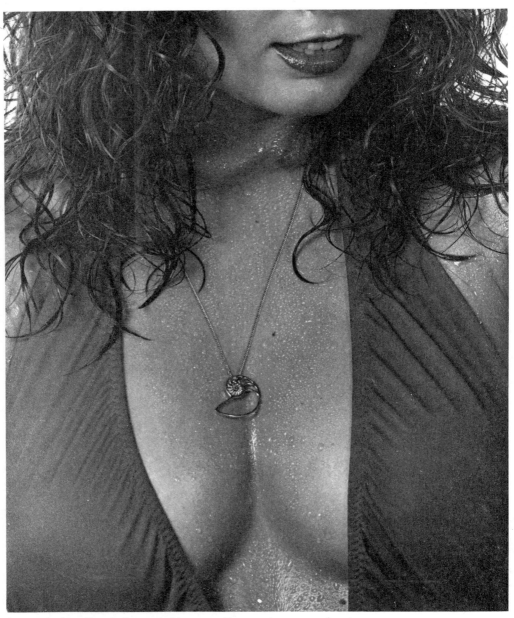

Accept the Nautilus challenge and become slimmer, stronger, and sexier.